D0849779

WILLIAM F. MAAG LIBRARY
YOUNGSTOWN STATE UNIVERSITY

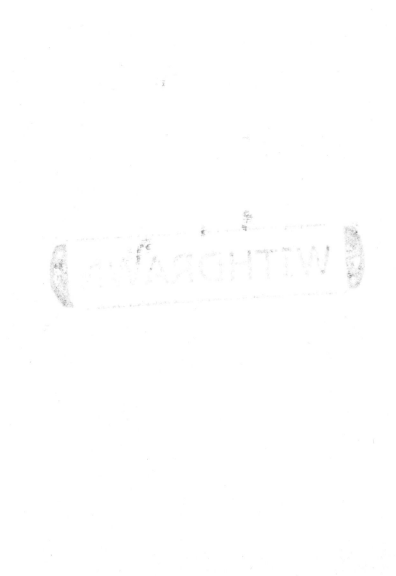
WITHDRAWN

Medicine and Society in France

Medicine and Society in France

Selections from the

Annales

Economies, Sociétés, Civilisations

Volume 6

Edited by

Robert Forster

and

Orest Ranum

Translated by

Elborg Forster

and

Patricia M. Ranum

The Johns Hopkins University Press
Baltimore and London

This book has been brought to publication with the
generous assistance of the Andrew W. Mellon Foundation.

Copyright © 1980 by The Johns Hopkins University Press

All rights reserved. No part of this book may be
reproduced or transmitted in any form or by any means,
electronic or mechanical, including photocopying,
recording, xerography, or any information storage and
retrieval system, without permission in writing
from the publisher.

Manufactured in the United States of America

The Johns Hopkins University Press, Baltimore, Maryland 21218
The Johns Hopkins Press Ltd., London

Library of Congress Catalog Card Number 79-16851
ISBN 0-8018-2305-6 (hardcover)
ISBN 0-8018-2306-4 (paperback)

Library of Congress Cataloging in Publication data
will be found on the last printed page of this book.

Contents

v

R
505
.H43

WILLIAM F. MAAG LIBRARY
YOUNGSTOWN STATE UNIVERSITY

Introduction

Health care touches every aspect of life. From the dangers for both mother and baby in childbirth to the illnesses of growing up and work, to epidemic diseases, to illnesses associated with poor diet and aging, and to ministering to the dying, individuals seek help as the pain and dangers to life threaten to overcome them. Nothing can be more social than health care; nothing could have more fundamental cultural, philosophical, and religious implications than society's response to those of its members who call for help because of the biological process itself, sickness, or accidents.

Hôtels-Dieu; hospitals for the sick; hospitals for the vagrant, orphan, and prostitute; and hospices, quacks, midwives, faith healers, physicians, surgeons, barbers, and nursing nuns made up the institutional and professional medical help that was available in preindustrial France. Together they responded to the appeals for their services, at once competing and arguing with each other for the right to help the sick as ordained by social custom and law. And, of course, there was competition for the payments made to them not only by the sick but by philanthropists and the state. The business side of health care reveals something of the aims and needs of the specific health care institutions and professions, such as the physicians and surgeons, whose income and status depended upon the esteem for their persons and services expressed by society. The history of the health care they offered is in its infancy. More is known about the pioneers in medicine and surgery, with their "breakthroughs" in health care, than about the routine care offered by the small town physician or the advice given by a quack. More is known about the civil servants who insisted that midwives be better trained than about the actual competence of the midwives themselves. Still less well known are the healers who lived down the path, it seems, in virtually every town and parish and who advised the wearing of copper bracelets to reduce rheumatic pains.

Encompassing not only the history of medicine and surgery, the history of health care has been defined in its broadest sense by scholars who have recently published on the subject in the *Annales.* What prompted the French to resort to quacks and to put up with what was often fatal advice about cures even through the nineteenth century? Answers to this question are partly supplied by Jean-Pierre Goubert as he finds that, while the physicians and surgeons made great claims to be the only "scientific" providers of health care, in fact, the society, through local authorities such as town councils and seigneurs, often protected those whom the doctors scorned as quacks. Why? Cultural and social reasons, to be sure, but also the high probability of failure to provide cures by both the "scientific" provider of health care and the quack. Even kings with their especially appointed physicians would occasionally try out remedies proposed by charlatans as they lay at death's door. Specialized functions for physicians enhanced their prestige; their Latin impressed the sick for centuries. But those whom they detested, the quacks, were given something akin to legal status thanks to community support and royal supervision.

The quarrels between the doctors and the quacks—and the quarrels between doctors and nursing nuns—are explored by Jacques Léonard. They remind us of the fuzzy boundary that separates the physicians from the chiropractors in our own day. Health care innovations trickled down from "scientific" medicine to the more popular practitioners. Goubert and Léonard together reveal how physicians were the first to be won over to Enlightened ideas about the influence of air and hygiene on health, only to be followed by the nursing nuns and eventually a change in the meaning of sin.

Marie-France Morel summarizes the discussion about the differing effects of city and country life on health care during the Enlightenment. Whatever was natural was thought to be better than what was artificial, and the natural prevailed in the country. City air was corrupted; doctors prescribed long stays in the country for their wealthier urban patients. Parents often made considerable financial sacrifices in order to permit a sickly child to grow up in the country. The analysis of body types to reveal different propensities to sickness and health would be combined with the effects on health of city and urban life in "scientific medicine." Only at the end of the eighteenth century did some medical writers begin to peer beyond ancient Greek medicine, or city/country and body type analyses to suggest more sophisticated modes of diagnosis.

Daniel Roche's study of the eulogies of physicians during the eighteenth century goes right to the heart of what the doctors thought they were doing for society and their strong sense of professionalism. Their attacks on miracle cures and quackery seem to put them in the vanguard of the scientific Enlightenment, at once antireligious and professional. In their eulogies of the colleagues who lost their lives while ministering to the sick in plague-ridden cities, however, the physicians formed a cult of sacrifice that lifted their roles in society to heights hitherto reserved for only martyrs and saints. The idea of the profession as a "calling" in the Weberian sense could apparently be made to conform with the teachings of Reason when tempered by martyrdom in helping the sick at the risk of the doctor's own life.

Along with the ambiguities and contradictions found in the health inspector's reports, Arlette Farge has unearthed some powerfully articulated social and economic presuppositions cloaked beneath humanitarian ideas. The inspectors were interested in increasing the docility of workers and their willingness to accept unpleasant and dangerous working conditions. There seems to be little emphasis on increasing productivity, however. Farge's research suggests that the royal health inspectors had only limited powers to intervene in the lives of artisan communities to alter manufacturing processes that were often centuries old. There was also a preoccupation with improving the quality of the air—that key to health according to "scientific medicine." In addition, a need for physical exercise was recognized by the inspectors. The nineteenth century would build upon this as a foundation for "moral improvement" in the belief that a clean, vigorous body would assure a "clean" and moral mind.

Muriel Joerger's research presents a taxonomy of the health care facilities that were available throughout France in the late eighteenth century. The functions and locations of the various types of institutions not only reveal population densities but again the preoccupation of royal officials and physicians with the health and social conditions associated with urban life. Joerger's research proposes a greater emphasis on physical rather than moral care for the indigent as a result of the French Revolution.

Finally, Mireille Laget recounts the terrible prejudices about childbearing and the incompetence of most who attempted to help women in labor. Midwives with little or no skill, or worse, midwives who claimed to have more skill than they actually had, were slowly displaced by more competently trained midwives. The humanitarian impulses of the Enlightenment in alliance with the arrogant pretensions of the physicians provided the foundation for royal enforcement of reform. But like so many other features of health care in the centuries prior to our own, the results in lives saved and pain reduced may not have been considerable.

A distinguished historian of medicine was asked the following question one day by a student: "At what time in history did it become statistically safer and better to call a doctor to seek health care than not to call one?" The historian reflected a moment and replied, "About 1925." Through the reading of these articles we glimpse the heart-rending history of generations of individuals who did what they could in the face of illness: they sought help. Their history is a bit more familiar to us now, as are the often heroic and fruitless attempts to help them in preindustrial France.

Robert Forster
Orest Ranum

Medicine and Society in France

1

The Art of Healing:
Learned Medicine and
Popular Medicine
in the France of 1790

Jean-Pierre Goubert

At the end of the eighteenth century, the effectiveness of medicine[1]—whether preventive or therapeutic—was not the indubitable fact it is today but, rather, a goal to be pursued, despite certain advances that had recently been made. Recourse to the physician, the surgeon ("the poor man's physician"),[2] or the midwife remained the prerogative of a minority that asserted its enlightenment, even though a concerted effort was made by the medical elite and the royal government to train midwives or to provide care for the poor in times of "epidemic disease." For the most part, of course, the French population practiced self-medication; it also consulted quacks, bone-setters, and matrons, listened to ambulant charlatans, and followed the course of treatment prescribed by the sorcerer-healer of the village.

Although the enlightened physicians of the eighteenth century took much of their inspiration from Hippocrates and Galen, they had come to question the set patterns of their learned tradition and to stress the prime importance of firsthand observation. Yet one wonders whether they were also able to understand the practices of popular medicine and to grasp the causes of its expansion and increasingly broad appeal. In view of the profusion of written documents they felt obliged to pass on to posterity, and of their zeal in denouncing charlatanry, which they viewed (in the years around 1789) as one of the four evils afflicting the "art of healing,"[3] one might be carried along by their self-assurance and their unanimity. To decide this matter on the basis of concrete evidence, certain testimonies left by the physicians and surgeons of the time must be carefully analyzed. These testimonies are to be found in the

Annales, E.S.C. 30 (September-October 1977): 908-26. Translated by Elborg Forster.

replies to the official surveys made in 1786 and 1790 and form the documentary basis of the present study.[4]

The Expansion of "Charlatanry"

In a France that was 85 percent rural, the testimony of patented surgeons who knew the small towns and rural areas, often because they practiced there, appears to be trustworthy. Of some one hundred responses sent (in 1790-91) from the four corners of the kingdom upon the request of the *Comité de Salubrité*[5] by the deputies of the king's first surgeon* and—though more rarely—by the surgeons' guilds, only six (6.2 percent) declared that they knew nothing of either "charlatans," "empirics," or "purveyors of nostrums" (*gens à secret*) within their district—which does not mean, of course, that there weren't any! Excepting these (as well as six evasive) responses, the statements considered here can be divided into three, numerically roughly equal, groups: 27 percent of the surgeons felt that the incidence of charlatanry was very high, 32.2 percent that it was high, and 28 percent that it was low. Under these circumstances, one must look into the attitudes of the observers. Their responses did not vary according to any precise geographical pattern (such as northern France versus southern France). In other words, one can come to only one conclusion: three different attitudes concerning the incidence of charlatanry prevailed among the patented surgeons, although it should be kept in mind that in almost 60 percent of the responses analyzed that incidence was considered to be high or very high—that is, too high—by the surgeons. Moreover, even the 34 percent of the respondents who felt that the incidence of charlatanry was low or even nonexistent unanimously denounced it anyway.

One additional indication of the significance—not in statistical but in symbolic terms—that must be given to these percentages is mentioned in some of the statements. The deputy-surgeon at Saint-Sever was the only one courageous enough to hand in a list of some fifty "empirics" and charlatans within his district, "not counting the priests who distribute aillot powders† and other unknown remedies."[6] As for the deputy surgeon of Luxeuil, he insisted on the role played by the "purveyors of nostrums, who are so well tolerated in this district that there is not one village without three or four persons who sell medicine. . . ."[7] The same view, the same image, is also given for the region of Josselin by the physician Lebard: "There is only one physician in the entire district of Josselin. Unless I am wrong, everyone is a physician: there is no one, of either sex, who does not meddle with giving advice to the sick, prescribing for them, or forbidding them to accept the most essential treatment and the most energetic remedies used in medicine."[8]

---

*For the sake of brevity, *lieutenant du premier chirurgien du roi* has been translated as "deputy surgeon" throughout.—Trans.

†Dr. Caroline Hannaway tells me that *poudre d'aillot* must refer to an antivenereal drug invented by Ailhaud and widely sold under the name "poudre d'Ailhaud."—Trans.

Just where did charlatanry begin? How can it be defined with any certainty? This raises the problem of stating the differences separating the nonmedical therapeutists from their officially certified colleagues. As far as the surgeons' discourse is concerned, the answer to this problem was perfectly clear. Charlatans? Why, they are people who illegally practice the art of healing. Seen in this manner, the outline presented by the surgeons reflects the culture-bound image of charlatanry held by the French medical profession at the end of the Ancien Régime, an image that was shared by the elite of physicians and the elite of surgeons, thus marking their fundamental kinship.

For this reason it is important to stress the mythical character of the opposition between learned and popular medicine.[9] If there was really a break between these two arts of healing, it was to be found at the end of the eighteenth century more at the level of collective notions than in the area of medical learning and social practice. In this respect, medicine was one, for all of its diversity and even its cleavages, except perhaps in the minds of the several thousand men who shared the social views of the Enlightenment.[10] In fact, these two "worlds" of medicine were so close to each other that they were in constant contact, both hating and penetrating each other. For one and the same patient might well turn successively or simultaneously to a physician, to a surgeon, and also to his healer—to the Devil but also to the Lord.[11]

Consequently, the questions asked of the representatives of the surgical profession by the Comité de Salubrité tell us something about the manner in which these men perceived the so-called popular medicine. Under these circumstances it would be absurd (even if it were possible) to try to measure the extension or the actual density of the network of charlatans. It would mean to accept the question asked in 1790 by the members of the Comité de Salubrité as entirely valid, without recognizing the fact that the committee transferred to a realm where it was not applicable a question that was valid for a preselected population, namely, the officially certified practitioners.

Actually, the question had been asked earlier by the controller general's office of the provincial administrators in a survey of 1786. This survey attempted to ascertain the medical statistics of the country as a whole and to assemble information concerning the professional quality of its physicians, surgeons, and midwives. The statistical analysis of the results of this survey concerning the physicians and surgeons (especially the latter), within the limits of northern France, leads to the following conclusion:[12] if the vast majority of the French population, especially in rural areas, only rarely consulted a physician or a certified surgeon, it was not because the medical network was lacking in density. In other words, the "medical desert" evoked by certain correspondents of the Société Royale de Médecine does not correspond to the actual facts; it only expresses—and this is not surprising—the refusal of an elite to include in the medical profession the masses of "second string" surgeons and popular therapeutists. The success of "charlatanry" in the France of 1780-90 was indeed a matter of concern to the medical profession of that period; especially the success of the category of surgeons who regularly treated a more rural, less "enlightened," and generally more modest clientele than their colleagues, the physicians.

Physicians and Charlatans

How, then, could a well-designed "medical policy" fail to ensure the future of the profession and also bring relief to a suffering humanity? The physicians' discourse, whether in 1790, around 1900, or even after 1970, constantly expresses the same obsession: "to confound [sic] charlatanry and bring enlightenment to so useful an art. . . ."[13]

In any case, and with respect to the late eighteenth century, the social border between "physician" and "charlatan," between learned and "popular" medicine, was not clearly drawn, however shocking this may seem to us. A few examples will briefly demonstrate this fact. The first set of testimonies is taken from the responses to the survey of the Comité de Salubrité concerning the practice of surgery (1790); the second comes from the survey of the kingdom's physicians and surgeons the intendants were ordered to conduct by the controller general's office in 1786.

At Montdidier the deputy surgeon reported "a charlatan admitted to the surgeons' guild." The deputy surgeon at Lyons-la-Forêt thundered against two "charlatans" who wanted to join the surgeons' guild.[14] Better yet, the deputy surgeon of Tonnère notes among the "empirics" "only one or two experts in urine, although they are not masters of surgery."[15] At Domfront, the deputy surgeon declared, speaking of "charlatans, empirics, and purveryors of nostrums": "there are many of them here, . . . even a physician and a surgeon who judge their patients' water by sight and give them medications from behind."[16]

For their part, the subdelegates who responded to the survey of 1786 often evoked the same problem. Thus, in speaking of the physician Lemaire, the subdelegate of Le Mans noted: "Was an empiric and does not enjoy the confidence of the public because of his passion for wine."[17] About the surgeon Lescot, a member of the guild in Saint-Georges-de-Ballon: "Was a charlatan selling drugs on the stage."[18] In the same manner the surgeon Lamour, in the subdelegate's opinion, was an "empiric [who] obtained permission to practice surgery and was admitted to the guild without being qualified."[19]

Yet in the survey of 1786 as a whole, the subdelegates rarely judged the surgeons so severely. Most of them simply counted and did not (or did only in veiled terms) express their opinion as to the professional quality of the surgeons they listed. But what shocked the local representatives of the central government was the incompatibility between a man's *incompetence* (that is, the lack of training received in a place recognized by the authorities) and the fact that he was granted the title of surgeon, even if, in practice, it amounted to no more than being master of surgery "having passed the *légère expérience*"* as stipulated for rural practitioners in the edict of Marly of 1707 and upheld in the version of 1772. This ambiguity was equally shocking to the deputy surgeons in their respective districts. This is no doubt why they blamed their predecessors, whom they considered to have been less particular, for admitting this or that charlatan. Thus, it was noted that in the countryside around Montdidier there was a "dangerous charlatan, admitted by my predecessor who was surgeon here in 1761, . . . and three bonesetters admitted contrary to the rules, long ago. . . ."[20] Similarly, in the area of Bray-sur-Seine, the local deputy surgeon notes the case of a shepherd admitted as a "bonesetter" in 1761.[21] In this manner the surgeons claimed that admitting empirics to the surgeons' guilds was done only in the past. But this does not mean that the number of empirics admitted between 1760 and 1790 was lower. Another hypothesis is equally plausible: The masters of surgery projected into the past an attitude they considered lax and reprehensible. And on the only occasion (out of some one hundred statements) when a surgeon speaks about this matter in the present tense, he does so in order to point out that at Nevers "empirics are not admitted."[22]

The deputy surgeon at Tartas (Landes) sums up rather well the image of these empirics held by the patented surgeons; empirics looked to them rather like the barber-surgeons, who, one would think, belonged only to the seventeenth century: "Few of them have had the necessary schooling, or even attended a college to take courses. Most of them become surgeons by chance. They have learned to wield a lancet. They consider some drug to be a full medical treatment. They move into a parish without any other training. . . ."[23] In responding to the survey of 1786, a number of subdelegates also stated that such surgeons only know how to "bleed and purge," or sometimes "shave and bleed."

Whether admitted to a surgeons' guild or not, these "surgeons-empirics" appear to have been very numerous in rural France in 1790. And yet, if we are to believe the statements analyzed here, they were actually on the side of the patented surgeons and physicians, for they "borrowed" or sought official recognition, practiced a "natural" medicine based on bleeding, purging, emetics, and simple or composite remedies, and followed—albeit from a distance—the sociocultural model imposed from "above." Thus, the official surgeons found themselves in an understandable quandary: should they reject these semisurgeons, or should they try to absorb them? Officially, of course, the outcome was rejection, expressed again and again in the various royal edicts and declarations, in the name of *competence* and with a view to the *monopoly* over which henceforth the medical profession wanted to keep full

---

*The *légère expérience* is explained in Toby Gelfand, "Medical Professionals and Charlatans,' the Comité de Salubrité Enquête of 1790-91," *Histoire Sociale-Social History* 11 (May 1978): 71-72.

control with the help of diplomas. This is why most of the deputy surgeons were distressed at their "inability to curb the country's empiricism. . . ."[24]

The unanimity and ferocity with which the surgeons lashed out against their colleagues the "semisurgeons" are all the more understandable as the latter took many patients away from them, thereby threatening their livelihood and diminishing the practices of those who, often of modest origin, had been obliged to pay for their education, examinations, and admissions fees. This is shown by published research on Anjou and Brittany, and it is confirmed by a broader study on the national scale, showing the levels of density of surgeons in the *généralités* of northern France for the towns and the rural areas.

These studies show that the potential clientele of the surgeon (and of the physician as well) was not very considerable, nor even elastic, despite the demographic growth of eighteenth-century France. The existence of two cultures, the patients' need to trust their therapeutist, the existence of a "wall of money"—all of this contributed to making the ascendancy of the official medical profession much less extensive than it considered desirable. And it is because they sensed—not too clearly at times—the importance of such obstacles to their advancement that the patented physicians and surgeons avidly seized the opportunity held out to them by the state to be recognized as the obligatory source of help and as the sole "specialists" in human sickness. This explains to a large extent their crusade against "empirics," "charlatans," and "purveyors of nostrums."

The Image of the Charlatan in Medical Circles

The analysis of 104 responses sent to the Comité de Salubrité enables us to see with somewhat greater precision the ideas about charlatanry that were current among surgeons. It is remarkable that no surgeon failed to answer the fourteenth and last question asked in the survey on "the practice of surgery in the kingdom."[25] In this connection, two complementary remarks are in order. The impact of the terminology proposed by the Comité de Salubrité proved to be considerable. In 41 percent of the responses analyzed, the proposed distinction among "charlatans," "empirics," and "purveyors of nostrums" was simply overlooked, and no comments were made. In other words, in 43 responses (out of 102), the patented surgeons refused to distinguish among three categories and lumped all of them together in an anonymous and vengeful "they." The anger of the patented surgeons prevented them from answering the question properly; in 41 percent of the cases the answer is limited to a plain statement: the charlatan is the other fellow!

Beyond this first assertion, however, the rest of the responses analyzed (59 percent of the total) are richer in nuances and information. In this group it is possible to present different aspects of the image of the "charlatan" held by 77 representatives of the surgical profession.

A closer look reveals that the majority of the surgeons (47 percent) denounced, first of all, the *itinerant* charlatans, but also those with a fixed residence, the "empirics" and "purveyors of nostrums." Among the settled charlatans were the "traditional village healers,"[26] and here the bonesetters occupied a prominent place. In fact, certain surgeons' guilds had admitted them and recognized their existence,[27] to the keen regret of the surgeons of 1790, who already favored an unqualified monopoly. This, whether they admitted it or not, was the reason why they excluded the bonesetters from their guild.

The other practitioners cited (see table 1.1)—dentists, oculists, hernia experts, pedicurists—were excluded in a similar manner. The surgeons treated them as a kind of subcategory of the paramedical type, thus foreshadowing the official medicalization of these occupations and their eventual inclusion in the health professions.

In the second rank of the accused we find the representatives of charitable medical organizations. For the most part, these were ecclesiastics, the majority of them regular clergy, primarily—as one would expect—nuns, and the Gray Sisters in particular. Better tolerated as a group in consideration of their "estate," they were nonetheless almost always designated as empirics, even

Table 1.1—Gamut of "Charlatans," According to the Words Used by Surgeons (77 Statements)

Stated Category	Number of References	Percentage of Total
Charlatans and healers		
Bonesetters	11	
Dentists	6	
Oculists	5	
Hernia specialists	4	
Spice mongers	3	
Pedicurists	2	
Straighteners	2	
Redresser	1	
Restorer	1	
Total	35	47%
Representatives of charitable medical organizations		
Nuns	10	
Secular clergy	8	
Monks	3	
Lay persons	2	
Total	23	30%
Members of the medical profession		
surgeons	13	
apothecaries	3	
physicians	2	
Total	18	23%
	Total	100%

WILLIAM F. MAAG LIBRARY
YOUNGSTOWN STATE UNIVERSITY

charlatans, and sometimes as purveyors of nostrums "of the worst kind." Such statements mark the dividing line that was supposed to separate those whose professional concern was with the body and with health from those whose professional concern was with the soul, with poverty, and with charity. It was, of course, in the name of the Enlightenment, in the name of their professional competence, and in the interest of the common good that the patented surgeons of 1790 rebelled against the interference of these "benefactors of the poor."[28]

Lastly, the deputy surgeons leveled charges of charlatanry against certain of their colleagues, namely, in ascending order, physicians, apothecaries, and surgeons. To be exact, these accusations applied only to the more or less "empiric" "semisurgeons" of the countryside. The physicians and apothecaries, for their part, were accused of encroachment, that is, of the illegal practice of surgery.[29] This was no longer a matter of medical men lashing out against charlatans, but rather of infighting within the medical profession.

In the final analysis, the vocabulary used by the patented surgeons is remarkably narrow and confused: narrow to the extent that these surgeons perceived and designated the various types of charlatans in terms of their "enlightened" culture, and confused, since the term "charlatan," which in the surgeons' minds was highly charged with emotion, became a vengeful epithet used to encompass and to exclude. In other words, they did not seem to know what it meant.

The "charlatans" were thus considered, on the first count, as actual or potential criminals. According to the expressions of the surgeons' representatives, they constituted a "scourge of humanity" (Beaugency), a "poisonous horde" (Pau), a "[special] race (Mont-de-Marsan), and a "sect of cannibals" (Breteuil). The deputy surgeon of Tartas, steeped in physiocratic thinking, spelled out the meaning of this accusation: "charlatans and empirics contribute to the country's depopulation. . . ."[30] This accusation also frequently flowed from the pens of intendants and subdelegates in their responses to the survey of 1786 and appears in the correspondence concerning "epidemic diseases," although it was leveled more often against the matrons and "so-called wise women."* In this manner the charlatan, the empiric, and all nonprofessionals appeared to be eminently harmful, if we follow the opinions of the masters of surgery and physicians, who judged the learning of the "charlatans" totally irrational and more than inadequate, considering them "a separate race," "barbarians," and savages. It was in the name of a learned culture bent on asserting its superiority that the medical profession—and in this instance the surgeons in particular[31]—loudly voiced its claim to the monopoly of health care.

The second count of the accusation (mutilations, accidents caused by imprudence and incompetence) concretely expresses the grievances and the reproaches directed against the "charlatans" by the surgeons. The deputy

---

*Pun on the French term *sage-femme*=midwife.—Trans.

surgeon at Nuits (Côte-d'Or) wrote in this connection: "We have women and men, both in our town and in the surrounding countryside, who meddle with treating the sick and giving them remedies. . . . We even have a woman oculist, well-versed in producing one-eyed and blind people, as well as individuals who claim that they can straighten cripples."[32] At times some compassion is expressed for the "unfortunate ones who are *martyred* by the charlatans."[33] (See table 1.2.)

Table 1.2—Surgeons' Charges against "Charlatans" (Based on 84 Responses)

Accusations	Number of Responses
Simple malfeasance	
Crime	22
Breach of trust	19
Accident	16
Incompetence	7
Illegal competition	4
Theft	2
Compounded malfeasance	
On two counts	
Crime and breach of trust	8
Crime and incompetence	3
Breach of trust and incompetence	2
Breach of trust and illegal competition	1
Theft and crime	1
Theft and breach of trust	1
Theft and illegal competition	1
On several counts	
Crime, breach of trust, incompetence	2
Crime, breach of trust, incompetence, theft	1
Crime, breach of trust, illegal competition, theft	1
Total	91

Given their animosity and their lack of understanding, the surgeons had no qualms about piling up the crimes and acts of malfeasance with which they charged the "charlatans." The logic underlying their hatred seems to proceed as follows: (1) the charlatan is incompetent, for he has not studied; (2) since he is incompetent, the charlatan causes accidents or, worse, commits crimes; and (3) under these conditions, charlatans are "knaves who dupe the people, . . . swindlers in fact, who try to mislead others about their health." All this because the learning of charlatans and healers did not proceed from a rational logic, founded upon a specific set of therapeutic procedures that were already seen as the only "scientific" ones!

Who Was Held Responsible?

In painting this extremely somber picture of the unfortunate effects of "popular" medicine, the surgeons did not fail to assign the responsibility for such a situation, even though the Comité de Salubrité had not asked any questions to that effect.

The responses of the surgeons were a manifestation of their professional code of ethics and their political consciousness. They therefore assigned prime responsibility (75 percent of the cases) to the institutions of the Ancien Régime,[34] above all, the "former judicial system," whose high cost and excessive slowness they recalled; they also noted the total ineffectiveness of the courts,[35] the ill will of the "seigneurial judges,"[36] as well as of the "erstwhile judges of the presidial courts."[37] Some of the surgeons did not hesitate to accuse certain judges who, in their "leniency"(?) took charlatans under their protection, thus shielding them from the justice of the law.[38] (See table 1.3.)

Table 1.3 — Responsibility for Charlatanry

Accused	Number of Testimonies
Institutions	
Police	24
Judicial system	23
Law	1
"Erstwhile intendant"	1
Total	49
Régime	
Ancien Régime	
Police	16
Judicial System	23
Law	1
Intendant	1
New regime	8
Total	49
People	
Popular credulity	12
In towns 3	
In countryside 9	
Physicians' laxity	4
Ancien Régime 2	
New Régime 2	
Total	16

Considering the matter in this light, the surgeons felt that they were being victimized. In fact, they were victimized by their own attitude. What unquestionably did hamper them was one of the real obstacles to their "enlightened" culture, that is, a medicine of the ethnographic type, a popular wisdom about the body that was so close to them that they learned about it through their wives and children and were liable to misunderstand it. That is why the new regime, however new it was, was not spared the criticism of the established surgeons either: the "medical police" that was in the hands of the municipal governments was accused of laxness, indeed total ineffectiveness.

On this point, the deputy surgeon of Meaux expressed himself as follows: "In the *arrondissement* of this guild there is a very large number of charlatans, empirics, purveyors of nostrums, and others, all of whom used to be authorized by the former police, and who are favored even more by the new."[39] At Vitry-le-François, the deputy surgeon indignantly noted: "The municipality grants permissions and thus permits the advertising of remedies that are distributed by charlatans, which is totally against all regulations. . . ."[40] As for J. N. Pellieux, a "soldier-citizen" and deputy surgeon at Beaugency, he foresaw with astonishing accuracy the *"embourgeoisement"* of the physician and of medicine that was to take place in the course of the nineteenth century: "The prolonged state of inertia of the administration of justice, as well as the laxness and the lack of experience with the laws concerning us on the part of the municipal officials, have enabled the charlatans to reappear more boldly than ever. . . . The professionals whose zeal does not take any action do no more than groan in secret; and one can only devoutly hope that because of it they will not be weak-minded enough to regret the demise of the Ancien Régime. . . ."[41]

The "pessimism of Cabanis and Cantin"[42] was echoed in the observations and the grievances offered by a small number of surgeons. If we are to believe them, that "expected brigandage"[43] held sway in certain areas long before the Thermidorian reaction. But it is possible that their judgment reflected not the actual situation but a heightened sensitivity toward "charlatanry."

Yet in the responses analyzed here the surgeons do not place all the blame on the regime, old or new. They felt—and explicitly said so—that the fundamental cause of charlatanry was to be found in the "credulity of the people," which, according to their testimony (9 out of 12), was more widespread in rural areas than in towns. The surgeons of Strasbourg, for example, stated: "The people of the countryside are more credulous than those of the towns."[44] At Boiscommun and also at Cognac,[45] the deputy surgeon felt that this popular credulity was due to the lack of enlightened education. At Mont-de-Marsan the local deputy depicted "a people impressed by the marvellous, . . . devoid of the faculty of discernment,"[46] which for this reason is easily deceived by charlatans. Clearly, the various explanatory factors invoked by the provincial surgeons fit into the typical ideology of the adherents to the second Enlightenment. As we now know, these explanations did not correspond to the social realities in the specific area of literacy and primary education.[47] Most importantly, however, the explanatory schema itself, proposed by diploma-holding and city-dwelling surgeons, is unconvincing, for a culture does not have to be founded on a narrow or short-sighted rationalism.

Pursuing their analysis of charlatanry, some of the surgeons saw it as more than a breach of trust committed by one kind of swindler or another. The deputy surgeon of Saint-Omer wrote, "The people . . . like to be deceived."[48] According to the deputy surgeon of Tours, "It even seems that the wretched class derives a kind of satisfaction from being deceived. . . ."[49] The deputy surgeon of Beaufort came to the following conclusion: "And with a heavy heart, we say to ourselves: the public wants to be deceived. So be it!"[50] What more is needed to show the discouragement, or perhaps the conscious or unconscious wisdom, of the surgeons faced with a "new world," inhabited by "savages" who refused the benefits of the Enlightenment?

Finally, the surgeons whose responses are recorded have spoken of the deepest cause of their failure; but since they felt that they represented a rational, learned, and (therefore) superior culture, the only "true" culture, they were unable to carry their analysis very far. Here is one indication, found in the response sent by the surgeons' guild of Cognac: "The number of purveyors of nostrums is also very large. They talk of *chaple, vertaupe,* and a lot of other foolishness of this kind, which surely is not part of the *nomenclature of diseases. Chaple,* according to them, is any mucous tumor appearing anywhere on the body. Scrofulous humors are called *vertaupe* by them."[51] Here we have the expression of "two interpretations of the world, two systems . . . that had become more alien to each other than ever before."[52] These statements also manifest—notwithstanding the translation proposed by the "enlightened" surgeons—the dismissal of a popular nomenclature of diseases. At the very time when they asserted the need for observation unhampered by any preconceived system, the surgeons adamantly refused to consider a different language, a different body of knowledge, because they felt that these were tied to a "popular" culture inferior to their own.

And yet, according to the testimony of several surgeons, this popular "credulity" was fostered not only by individuals within the lower classes and by "vulgar" swindlers, but also—what dreadful treason!—by members of the medical profession. In this connection, the deputy surgeon of Vitry-le-François wrote, "The physicians give out certificates for which they charge, so that the public is misled. . . ."[53] As for the deputy of Nuits, he denounced "all the charlatans kept in business by the king's first physician, who, for a certain sum, gave them the power to commit murder everywhere in France for three years. . . ."[54] In this manner, the issue of nostrums (whose sale was permitted) revived an old quarrel between physicians and surgeons. Neither the activities of the Royal Commission of Medicine nor, later, those of the Royal Society of Medicine, the two bodies that were successively charged with policing these "secret remedies," were able to obviate this quarrel. In the years around 1760, for example, Charles Dionis, doctor-regent of the Faculty of Medicine of Paris (and grandson of the famous surgeon and anatomist Pierre Dionis), owned and operated the royal privilege concerning the sale of Orvietan, having bought it from the Contugi family. He charged the retailers of Orvietan high prices for their franchises and did not hesitate to have his children advertise this remedy on the stage.[55] Brother Côme, first physician to Louis XV, also upheld this lucrative tradition. And when the young Fabre d'Eglantine* was "driven to the wall by his creditors"[56] in 1789, he did not hesitate to become a "ghost writer" for the inventor of an antinephritic.

The surgeons' attitude toward "charlatanry" seems very passive: 52 percent simply recorded facts; 25 percent admitted their resignation; and only 23

---

*Fabre d'Eglantine later put his hand to the framing of the Revolutionary calendar.—Trans.

percent were in favor of "effective" repressive measures. And even among these 23 percent, we must deduct almost one-third who felt satisfied with the repressive measures carried out at the time; half of them concerning the repression of charlatanry in the towns and half of them concerning the severe repression carried out in the countryside.[57] (See table 1.4.)

Table 1.4—Surgeons' Attitudes toward Charlatanry

Item		Percentage of Responses
Attitudes recorded		
Statement of fact		52%
Resignation to charlatanry		25
Demands for repression		23
Total		100%
Analysis of repressive attitudes		
Satisfied with existing repressive measures		31%
In towns	50%	
In countryside	50	
Wishing for stronger repressive measures		69
In towns	10	
In countryside	90	
Total		100%
Modes of repression*		
Legislative mode		50%
By the law	33	
By the wisdom of the legislative assembly	17	
Constitutional mode		11
Corporatist mode		17
Total		100%

*The figures in this category appear incomplete.—Trans.

As for the surgeons who saw the solution in an intensified struggle against charlatanry, they either supported (in one-third of the cases) a "stable and wise law"[58] to be passed by the National Assembly, placed their trust in the "wisdom of the Assembly,"[59] or else counted on the "new Constitution" for the resolution of problems of this kind.[60] In other words, this "active minority," which considered itself a repository of the Enlightenment, placed its trust in the constitutional monarchy; above all, it felt that the unfortunate position of the medical profession in its opposition to charlatanry could be remedied by a law to be made by an assembly of enlightened individuals. This solution was a logical one for the men of the Enlightenment. Clearly, this minority of enlightened surgeons expected that it would be possible to change the ways of a "credulous populace" by a constant barrage of decrees, circulars, and punitive measures. One wonders whether we today must agree with them—not because they were right, but because of what has happened.

Under these circumstances, the "repressive" minority felt that the best solution would be to entrust the medical profession not only with its own internal governance but also with the policing of and the jurisdiction over the representatives of "charlatanry." The deputy surgeon of Mont-de-Marsan expressed himself as follows: "Some of them present themselves with such an air of importance, with false titles, and in such beguiling ways that the real professionals are almost the only ones not to be seduced by them. . . . And I know of no surer means of extirpating this race [sic] than to give the power to do so to the professionals."[61]

The comparison among the three approaches I have just outlined reveals two essential contradictions. On the one hand, the seriousness of the misdeeds with which the "charlatans" were charged contrasts with the passivity of the vast majority (75 percent of the responses analyzed) of the surgeons. Only a small minority was consistent with its own attitude and demanded sharper repressive measures. On the other hand, the criticism leveled against political institutions (above all the Ancien Régime, for a minority expected a great deal from the new one) by the surgeons is offset by a low "level of innovation": only 23 percent of the surgeons (in the sample analyzed) proposed measures that would, in their opinion, solve the problem of "charlatanry." However, the measures advocated by that minority, that is, the resort or return to restrictive regulations, implied that the New Regime would be more willing or able to break the "credulity of the populace" than the Ancien Régime. What contends against this possibility is the resigned or passive attitude of all the surgeons who had little faith in the application and the effectiveness of such regulatory texts.

These two contradictions in the attitudes of the enlightened surgeons are easily explained if one takes a closer look at their mentality. Their attitudes as "enlightened" men prevented them from understanding a culture different from their own; this is why they were unable to do more than note the facts and why, in the name of their principles, they limited themselves to judging and condemning. Some of them were vaguely aware that they were frustrated by something strange; and this either made them angry or fostered resignation, due to a political attitude of "wait and see" or to personal conviction.

Activities and Personal Characteristics of the "Charlatans"

Given the nature of the testimonies analyzed, one must be careful in presenting a "mug shot" of the accused. To begin with, the number of detailed descriptions taken from real life, as it were, turns out to be very small. This, of course, is not surprising, since such descriptions—which, when written by "enlightened" surgeons, were designed to specify the imbecility and the misdeeds peculiar to "charlatans"—were usually considered superfluous, for it is easiest to judge what one does not perceive!

In this manner, there are thirty-five descriptions (of at least one sentence) scattered throughout the approximately one hundred responses sent to the Comité de Salubrité and analyzed here. Of these thirty-five "descriptions," twenty-one concern ecclesiastics who were treated as empirics, that is—notwithstanding the good intentions for which they were given credit—as incompetent and therefore dangerous people. In addition, we have some fifteen brief descriptions, only one of them—a laconic statement—concerning a female charlatan.

In the urban world, several "corporations" [guilds] had, according to the surgeons' testimony, a special reputation for engaging in the (illegal) practice of medicine, surgery, and pharmacy, namely, the executioners, cabinet makers, and spice mongers. At Angoulême, for example, "the executioner of high justice sets fractures and sprains or pretends to set them. . . ."[62] At Narbonne, several cabinet makers engaged in dressing wounds and bleeding,[63] while at Quesnoy a mason played the role of dentist.[64] As for the spice mongers, despite the edict of August 1766 stipulating the separation between spice mongers and apothecaries, "they sold remedies at Bray-sur-Seine, often without knowing their effect and without a prescription from the professionals, spurred on by their desire for gain."[65] At Arras—and this case is far from unusual —another "specialty" was practiced by resident empirics. "One family, many of whose members practice surgery, has no other talents than that of operating on all inguinal hernias by castrating the patient."[66] Aside from these "specialized" empirics, it would seem, however, that many others played the role of veritable general practitioners; in particular the urban representatives of charitable medicine and, above all, the Gray Sisters.

For the rural world we find, in the writings of the surgeons, the same specialized empirics, the same medical and paramedical categories. In some cases the occupations of these men have changed; we still find blacksmiths and spice mongers, though we no longer find executioners but instead a number of ordinary peasants. In the rural Vendée, for example, near Vouvant-en-Chataigneraie, "the village's match peddlers sell leftover drugs from [drug] stores . . . at several times the price they have paid for them. . . ."[67] And at Meung-sur-Loire the blacksmith practiced the *"métier* of charlatan." Curiously he was designated successively, first as "charlatan," then as "empiric," and finally as "sorcerer" by the deputy surgeon of Beaugency. "Last year," the latter wrote, "a miller of Tavers near Beaugency went to *consult* him about his wife; upon inspection of the urine, the blacksmith declared that the woman was bewitched but that for 100 *écus* he would heal her. The gullible miller brought in the money; and a beef heart pierced with needles, a crucifix lying on its side, blessed candles, and a few words spoken in the miller's presence were the means by which he performed his operation. . . ."[68]

Among the one hundred testimonies analyzed, only one furnishes positive proof of the identity between the traditional healer and the sorcerer; this identity was also found by P.-Y. Sébillot, M. Bouteiller, and J. Favret in their research.[69] The difference between two conceptions of the world was both so tenuous and so pervasive that the "enlightened" surgeons were virtually unable to see the typical practices of "popular" medicine.

Lacking descriptive information about the practices of sorcery in the village, the enlightened surgeons identified a certain kind of charlatan and empiric as sorcerers, as is clearly indicated in two of the testimonies. Thus, one of the physicians of Hyères singled out as his favorite target "the purveyors of nostrums, especially those who impress the credulous people by pretending to be sorcerers. . . ."[70] The surgeons of Ustaritz considered the "charlatans" as "magicians of sorts."[71] The deputy surgeon at Saint-Sever (Landes) pointed to the shepherds, these quasi-mythological beings "who from the beginning of time have occupied a special place in the life of the peasants." But it is in the turning of a phrase that the opposition between two concepts of the world suddenly bursts forth; as when the informant rejects the notion of a universal remedy in favor of "specifics": "shepherds . . . come down from the mountain and stay with us as long as the winter lasts to guard their flocks in our cantons; and even in our town they peddle their cures, applying poultices and selling nostrums that they claim to be infallible against all ills."[72]

About itinerant—rather than transhuming—charlatans there is little information. Some of them came to town (or to the *bourg* [small market town]) on fixed dates, on the days when fairs or markets were held.[73] At Carcassonne it was the first Saturday of each month.[74] They "set up a stage on the public square" and "begin by entertaining the public"; this was done, for instance, by "a man named Aubry at Bellegarde."[75] Thereupon they advertise and sell "their drugs and their balms," their "purgative pills, poultices, herbs," and so forth. Certain others performed surgery, as at Bellegarde, or practiced medicine. Thus, at Auch—what a dreadful scandal!—"a man by the name of Toscan, . . . that charlatan, made people throw away the medicines prescribed by M. Cortade, the physician, and put the patients on his own medicines. . . ."[76] Elsewhere, itinerant charlatans advertised a specialty, operating as oculists or dentists, according to the testimony of the surgeons of Laon or Morlaix.

In this manner, the enlightened surgeons classified their competitors by the medical function they assigned to them. The pharmacist was the counterpart of the seller of "dangerous" drugs or the empiric; to the physician and the surgeon corresponded the specialists in the many ills of daily life (oculists, dentists, bonesetters) as well as the "generalists" who practiced sorcery or sold universal remedies. The enlightened surgeons made every effort to classify the practitioners of charlatanry in a logical and functional manner. In doing so they transferred to the domain of "popular" medicine a grid and a set of values that applied to the domain of learned medicine. Consequently, the classification they proposed enables us to measure certain deviations from the norm they hoped to enforce. Their vision of "charlatanry" reflects their concept of learned medicine.

The basic characteristic of all charlatans, empirics, and purveyors of nostrums, they felt, was the lack of competence of all the types they attempted to differentiate. This we must see as an unequivocal sign of the determination asserted by apothecaries, physicians, and surgeons, to see the practice of their art exclusively in the hands of the only profession that would provide every ethical and scientific guarantee. In this manner, they contrasted the "obscurantism" of the charlatans with the Enlightenment of "learned" medicine.[77] Having at their disposal a body of learning they considered superior, "enlightened" physicians and surgeons felt that they could not possibly commit any errors in the exercise of their art, and that it would be the exclusive prerogative of the "charlatans" to maim, murder, or deceive their patients! Yet, in the same manner as the "charlatan" who sold his "miracle" drugs, the physician who wanted to monopolize the health field collected—and this was only fair—his honoraria, just like a lawyer, a notary, or even certain academic teachers.

Still another area in which the analysis carried out by the surgeons reflects their vision of the medical profession is the minimal importance they attributed to women in their assessment of charlatanry. Minimal ideed, for the medical profession was not to grant a woman the degree of Doctor of Medicine until 1875! Even when it was only a matter of denouncing "charlatans," no more than three patented surgeons so much as broached the subject of women. Only the deputy surgeon at Luxueil noted that a majority of the "purveyors of nostrums" were women; on the other hand, the physician Lebard (resident of Josselin) and the deputy surgeon of Nuits estimated that in the rural areas the practice of charlatanry was shared equally between men and women. But only one of these three informants, the deputy surgeon at Nuits, betrayed his antifeminine attitude when he noted that among the purveyors of nostrums of his district there was "even one female oculist, well versed in producing one-eyed and blind people."[78]

Among the responses to the survey of 1786 (concerning patented physicians and surgeons), not one mentions a woman practicing medicine or surgery. In the responses to the survey on midwives (1786), one letter only, signed by two parish priests of the Médoc, points out and recommends "Madame Banny de Rey, master of surgery."[79] This laudatory statement is the only one to counterbalance, as it were, the mass of hostile observations characteristic, in the survey on midwives of 1786, of the physicians and surgeons who responded. Do we here touch the roots of a medical antifeminism that held sway for so long, and indeed to our own day?

The analysis of such a series of documents, finally, must cover more than the explicit statements. Certain omissions—particularly with repsect to the role of female therapeutists—raise questions about the nature of the couple and of the family, both nuclear and extended, and about the complex interaction of the roles played by both. Other omissions imply that the imputation of "sorcery" had become fused, at least to some extent, with that of "charlatanry." Sorcery seems to have become more secular in the years since the ordinance of 1682;[80] also, males seem to have become more involved in it, to the detriment of the traditional mouthpiece of the Evil One, the female!

Another omission is equally meaningful. None of the documents consulted —for the period 1780-90—breathes a single word about healing saints. It is not surprising, of course, that they had not yet gained recognition in official questionnaires. Do we therefore have to assume that "enlightened" administrators and physicians consciously avoided so delicate a subject? For it was delicate, involving as it did the difference between faith and credulity, between layman and ecclesiastic, between believers and unbelievers.

Omitted also was the so-called popular literature. Not one of the almanacs or medical pamphlets was condemned. Nor was anything said about the health care manuals or journals that experienced a considerable development at the time and were signed by, among others, a number of physicians and surgeons, sometimes under a false name. These were "paperbacks" that constituted, as they still do today, an important vehicle for the successful dissemination of hygienic measures of the learned type, that is, a necessary popularization of science in the best sense of the term.

The ultimate and most revealing omission concerns the issue of nostrums (*remèdes secrets*). The physicians and surgeons always approached it in terms of their principles and their professional code of ethics, which is why they always affirmed the principle of specialization and evoked the complementary functions of the physician who prescribed and the pharmacist who delivered the remedy, and why they also affirmed the principle that a remedy (and thus its formula, which was called "secret") belonged to its inventor or inventors, who exploited it under a privilege. (That privilege was to become a right after the Revolution, when the bourgeoisie came into its own.) In other words, one wonders whether the consumer, the client, the sick patient, the diseased living body and, by the same token, the problem of self-medication, were forgotten. As for the absence of information from medical sources about the nature of the "baneful secrets"* and about abortive procedures, it is not surprising either, for what could be more contrary in principle to the Hippocratic oath?

The analysis of the responses to the surveys of 1786 and 1790 has provided a series of revealing testimonies about the mentality of the French medical profession concerning the relationship between learned and "popular" medicine. It has brought to light certain problems of interpretation involved in reading a set of documents of learned origin and character. First of all, it confirms the assumption that the ideology of the Enlightenment had reached the group of masters of surgery as a whole as well as their urban elite. When it came to "charlatanry," their "discourse" deviated very little from that of the "enlightened" correspondents of the Société Royale de Médecine or of certain Parisian master apothecaries. The irresistible ascent of surgery and pharmacy in professional and scientific terms[81] was in part responsible for the establishment of closer ties between some of the surgeons and the physicians; it was a *rapprochement* that foreshadowed, albeit from afar, the eventual unification of the medical profession that was to take place in 1892.

The second testimony provided by the *corpus* examined here is this: better

---

*This was the contemporary euphemism for contraceptive practices. — Trans.

administrative techniques for taking a survey (which had been perfected in the course of the eighteenth century) tended to reinforce the preconceived notions of an elite that meant to stress its enlightenment. The medical elite also expressed, very forcefully indeed, its "will to power," its will to monopolize the vast field of health care, from which it excluded all nonprofessionals with a grim determination that was rooted in a centuries-old tradition and strengthened by the ideology of the Enlightenment.

Altogether, then, the medical elite clearly outlined the undertaking it was to pursue throughout the nineteenth and twentieth centuries, namely, a veritable crusade against charlatanry and a struggle to impose medical control upon the body social as a whole. During the 1780s a group of men, asserting their superiority, laid claim to the exclusive practice of an art that was itself considered the fruit of superior learning. This, among other things, explains the masculine image of the therapeutist in the discourse of the enlightened surgeons, not only on the level of the images projected (sorcerers were designated as such, but nothing was said about witches) but also on the level of social realities, as exemplified by the increasing numbers of physicians practicing obstetrics and surgeons demonstrating the techniques of delivery.

This was the attitude of a conquering power; it was also a lazy and ultimately unwarranted attitude, for it side-stepped the authentic problems raised by the existence of a popular culture, problems that must be faced by the historian as well as by the anthropologist or the physician. In our own time the scientific, professional, and social success of medicine and the medical profession is so great that in the present medical elite one can observe the reappearance of the feeling of superiority and the same self-assurance that pervades the enlightened texts of the eighteenth century. In order to stress the superiority of its learning, the medical profession has reduced or denied the veiled kinship, the mere nuance of difference, the sigh [of mutual attraction] that existed—and still exists—between "legitimate physicians and charlatans."[82] And this nuance is due not only to the increasing (and that means both dangerous and beneficial) effectiveness of medical knowledge, but also to two different systems of understanding the world. It also involves the matter of personal identity. As for the denial of this nuance, it "has its source in the peculiar relationships obtaining in the social and the natural order, where the first [group], once it has detached itself from the second, attains a sovereign position, thanks to mankind's adaptation to that segment that holds the tools"[83] of power.

Appendix

The circular letter (dated Paris, 24 November 1790, and signed by Drs. Guillotin and Gallet, respectively president and secretary general of the Comité de Salubrité) contains fourteen questions concerning the situation of surgery in the kingdom. Only questions 12 and 14 relate directly to "popular medicine."

Question 12: "Are other practitioners admitted separately, under such special designations as dentists, oculists, hernia experts, bonesetters, pedicurists, etc.?"

Question 14: "Are charlatans, empirics, and purveyors of nostrums [*gens à secret*] very prevalent in your district? To what extent are they tolerated?"

NOTES

1. According to Monthyon, it was still an open question "whether medicine destroys more people than it saves." Cited in Pierre Goubert, *Histoire économique et sociale de la France* (Paris, 1970), 2: 65.

2. Archives départementales (hereafter A.D.), Aisne, C 19; Soissons, 1 October 1786, Intendant's report to the Controler-General on the physicians and surgeons of his generality.

3. Michel Foucault, *Naissance de la clinique* (Paris, 1963), p. 44; [English translation by A. M. Sheridan Smith, *Birth of the Clinic* (New York, 1973)]. See also Jean-Pierre Peter, "Malades et maladie," *Annales, E.S.C.* (July-August-September 1967): 711-51 [English translation in R. Forster and O. Ranum, eds., *Biology of Man in History* (Baltimore: The Johns Hopkins University Press, 1975), pp. 81-124]; J.-P. Peter, "Les Mots et les objets de la maladie," *Revue historique* 499 (July-September 1971): 38.

4. On the survey of 1786, see J.-P. Goubert and F. Lebrun, "Médecins et chirurgiens dans la société française du XVIIIe siècle," *Annales cisalpines d'histoire sociale* 4 (1973): 119-36. For an approach on the regional level, cf. F. Lebrun, *Les Hommes et la mort en Anjou (Paris-The Hague, 1971), pp. 199 ff; cf. also J.-P. Goubert, Malades et médecins en Bretagne . . .* (Paris, 1974), pp. 78 ff. Another series of documents on "secret remedies" (the papers of the Société Royale de Médecine) has been analyzed by Matthew Ramsey (forthcoming).

5. This is the survey launched by the Comité de Salubrité, a survey calling for declarative statements and sent in the form of a circular letter dated 24 November 1790 to the deputies of the king's first surgeon. The circular letter contained fourteen questions concerning "the practice of surgery in the kingdom," with two of the questions relating directly to the representatives of "popular" medicine; cf. the suggestive wording of these questions in the appendix to the present study. For this survey of the Comité de Salubrité, see also H. Ingrand, *"Le Comité de Salubrité de l'assemblée nationale constituante (1790-91),"* (Thesis in medicine, University of Paris, 1934); see also M.-J. Imbault-Huart, "Sources de l'histoire de la médecine aux archives nationales de 1750 à 1822," *Revue d'histoire des sciences* 25 (January-March 1972): 51-52. In the present study, I am using cartons F¹⁵ 226-228(2), which had been studied by Henri Ingrand, and F¹⁷ 2276 of the National Archives. Other responses to the same survey (not analyzed here) can be found in series L of departmental archives.

6. Archives nationales (hereafter A.N.), F¹⁷ 2276, item 334b. The district of the deputy surgeon at Saint-Sever corresponded, as it was customary at the time, to the jurisdiction of the bailliage court of the same name. This was before the kingdom had been divided into departments.

7. A.N., F¹⁷ 2276, item 336, Luxeuil, 15 January 1791.

8. Ibid., item 269b, Josselin, 22 January 1791.

9. Cf., by contrast, the thesis concerning the nature of "popular" medicine defended by L. Boltanski in *La Découverte de la maladie* (Paris, 1968), 1: 23ff.

10. Cf. Peter, "Les Mots et les objets de la maladie."

11. Cf. J.-C. Souria, *Mythologie de la médecine moderne* (Paris, 1969), p. vii: "No less than the peasants, engineers in electronics and graduates of the Ecole Polytechnique frequent charlatans and bonesetters, people who swing the pendulum, peer into the patient's iris, and weigh his hair. . . ."

12. For the density of the medical network in France, 1780-90, cf. Lebrun, *Les Hommes et la mort en Anjou,* pp. 199 ff.; Goubert, *Malades et médecins en Bretagne,* pp. 78-119; also Goubert and Lebrun, "Médecins et chirurgiens." For the nineteenth century, I refer the reader to Jacques Léonard's "Les Médecins de l'Ouest au XIXe siècle" (Doctoral thesis, University of Paris-I, 1976) and to Jean Waquet's forthcoming article on the ventôse law of the year XI [1803]. For the period 1780-90, cf. J.-P. Goubert, "The Extent of Medical Practice in France about 1780," to be published in a special issue of *Journal of Social History.*

13. A.D., DXXXVIII, session of the conseil de Santé, 15 ventôse, year III. Cf., on the same issue, the royal declaration of 25 April 1777, creating the Royal College of Pharmacy in Paris.

14. A.N., F[17] 2276, item 288, Lyons-la-Forêt, n.d. [December 1790].

15. Ibid., item 349, Tonnerre, 23 January 1791. On the examiners of urine, cf. C. Guyot-jeannin, "Contribution à l'histoire de l'analyse des urines" (Thesis in pharmacy, University of Strasbourg, Creteil, 1951).

16. A.N., F[17] 2276, item 307, Domfront, 5 January 1701. "Judging the water by sight": the consultant looks at the urine, lifting the vessel containing it up to eye level. As for "giving remedies to the patients from behind," I propose that this expression be taken quite literally. In this case it would mean treatment by means of enemas, for example.

17. A.D., Indre-et-Loire, C 354, Le Mans, 1786.

18. Ibid.

19. Ibid., C 354, subdelegation of Beaumont-la-Vicomté, 1786.

20. A.N., F[15] 228[2], item 3, Montdidier, 30 November 1790.

21. Ibid., item 7, Bray-sur-Seine, 2 December 1790.

22. A.N., F[17] 2276, item 347[a], Nevers, 11 February 1791, report of Bonnet, epidemic surgeon.

23. A.N., F[17] 2276, item 342, Tartas, 20 January 1791. The same opinion, the same "discourse," the same confusion among charlatans, empirics, and purveryors of nostrums is to be found in the *Dictionnaire de Trévoux* (Paris, 1743), vol. 2, col. 1693, s.v. "empirique," and ibid., vol. 1 col. 1995, s.v. "charlatan." Cf. also, in the same vein, the article "charlatan," written by the Chevalier de Jaucourt, in the *Encyclopédie* (Paris, 1753), 3: 208-10.

24. A.N., F[17] 2276, item 342, Tartas.

25. Cf. below, the text of this question no. 14 in the appendix to the present article.

26. M. Bouteiller, *Médecine populaire d'hier et d'aujourd'hui* (Paris, 1966), p. 46.

27. In this connection, cf. Dr. E. Olivier, *Médecine et santé dans le pays de Vaud au XVIIIe siècle (1675-1798)* (Lausanne, 1962), 1: 422 ff.

28. Bouteiller, *Médecine populaire*, p. 26. Cf., in the same vein, paragraph 8 of the royal declaration of 28 April 1777.

29. A.N., F[17] 2276, item 266, Angoulême, competition between apothecaries and physicians; ibid., item 331, Bergerac, competition from physicians. It should be pointed out that physicians were authorized to practice *propharmacie* in districts that lacked an established pharmacist.

30. Ibid., item 294, Nuits, 29 December 1790. Cf. below, note 65.

31. Cf., in the same vein, the address given for the inauguration of the royal College of Pharmacy on Monday, 30 June 1777 by one of its provosts, the master apothecary Trevez; Archives of the Ecole de Pharmacie, register A 39, pp. 8 ff.

32. Ibid.

33. A.N., F[17] 2276, item 304, Parthenay.

34. The expression "Ancien Régime" appears in the responses sent by the surgeons of Beaugency and Morlaix. It is also frequent in the *Cahiers de doléances* written by the apothecaries, surgeons, and physicians. Cf. D. Lorillot, *"Essai sur les cahier de doléances des médecins, chirurgiens et apothicaires en 1789"* (Master's thesis, University of Paris-I, 1975). (This is a sampling of eight provincial towns.)

35. A.N., F[17] 2276, item 303, Morlaix, 17 January 1791.

36. Ibid., item 342, Tartas.

37. Ibid., item 354, Ustaritz.

38. Ibid., F[15] 228[2], Montereau. Similar observations can be found in the case of Ussel (ibid., F[17] 2276, item 300) and Poitiers (ibid., item 293).

39. Ibid., F[15] 228[2], item 10, Meaux, 3 December 1790.

40. Ibid., F[17] 2276, item 281, Vitry-le-François, 28 December 1790.

41. Ibid., F[15] 227[1], Beaugency, 1 December 1790.

42. Foucault, *Naissance de la clinique*, p. 64. In this connection see also J. Léonard, "L'Exemple d'une catégorie socio-professionnelle au XIXe siècle: Les Médecins français," in *Ordes et classes: Colloque d'histoire sociale, Saint-Cloud, 24-25 mai 1967* (Paris-The Hauge, 1973), pp. 221 ff. Also J. Léonard, "Les Médecins de l'Ouest au XIXe siècle" (Doctoral thesis, University of Paris-I, 1976. See, furthermore, the texts concerning the physician as notable assembled by Louis Bergeron in *Annales, E.S.C.* 32 (September-October 1977): 863-65.

43. Foucault, *Naissance de la clinique*, p. 45.

44. A.N., F[17] 2276, item 359.

45. Ibid., items 278 and 337.

46. Ibid., item 357.

47. Cf. the collective study of the Centre de Recherches Historiques directed by F. Furet and J. Ozouf; also of interest, M. de Certeau, D. Julia, and J. Revel, *Une Politique de la langue: La Révolution française et les patois* (Paris, 1975), pp. 137 ff.

48. A.N., F^{17} 2276, item 351.

49. Ibid., item 330.

50. Ibid., item 339.

51. Ibid., item 278, Cognac.

52. M. Crubellier, *Histoire culturelle de la France* (Paris, 1974), p. 89.

53. A.N., F^{17} 2276, item 281.

54. Ibid., item 294. The deputy surgeon of Nuits alluded to the ruling of the king's council of 17 March 1731.

55. Cf. Le Paulmier, *L'Orviétan* (Paris, 1892), pp. 95-107.

56. According to Joël Fouilleron, "Fabre d'Eglantine et les chemins du théâtre," *Revue d'histoire moderne et contemporaine* 21 (July-September 1974): 503.

57. Cf. J.-P. Peter, "Le Grand Rêve de l'ordre médical, en 1770 et aujourd'hui," *Autrement* 4 (1975/76): 183-92.

58. A.N., F^{17} 2276, item 330, Tours.

59. Ibid. item 316, Auch.

60. Ibid., item 334, Saint-Sever.

61. Ibid., item 357, report signed by "the provost of the community of masters of surgery of Mont-de-Marsan (Landes), writing in the name of the community."

62. Ibid., item 266. Cf., for this issue, M.-A. Saint-Léger, "Conflit entre le corps des chirurgiens et le bourreau de Lille en 1768," *Revue du Nord* 2 (1911): 49.

63. A.N., F^{17} 2276, item 274.

64. A.N., F^{15} 228^1, Le Quesnoy (Nord).

65. A.N., F^{15} 228^2, item 7, 2 December 1790.

66. A.N., F^{17} 2276, item 312. Other examples of castrations of this kind are found in two subdelegates' responses to the survey of 1786 and in A.D. Eure, 5 M 1, item 1, 19 brumaire an V [1797].

67. A.N., F^{17} 2276, item 353, undated. For a comparison with today, cf. Andrè Burguière, *Bretons de Plozévet* (Paris, 1975) and Pierre Jakez Hélias, *Le Cheval d'orgeuil* (Paris, 1975).

68. A.N., F^{15}, 227, Beaugency, 1 December 1790, response by J.-N. Pellieux, deputy of the king's first surgeon.

69. Cf. P.-Y. Sébillot, *Le Folklore de la Bretagne* (Paris, 1968), 1: 151; also M. Bouteiller, *Sorcier et jeteurs de sort* (Paris, 1957); idem, *Médecine populaire;* J. Favret, "Le Malheur biologique et sa répétition," *Annales, E.S.C.* 26 (May-August 1971): 873-88; M. Foucault, "Les Déviations religieuses et le savoir médical," in *Hérésies et sociétés* (Paris-The Hague, 1968), pp. 19-29.

70. A.N., F^{17} 2276, item 33^b, Hyères, 20 February 1791.

71. Ibid., item 354, 24 January 1791. Cf. R. Mandrou, *Magistrats et sorciers en France au XVIIIe siècle* (Paris, 1968), p. 456.

72. A.N., F^{17} 2276, item 334^a, Saint-Sever, 20 January 1791. For the "meeting" between universal remedy and specific remedies, see the remarkable master's thesis (University of Paris-I) by Pascale Muller, "Les Eaux minérales en France à la fin du XVIIIe siècle" (1975).

73. This was a case at Le Quesnoy (A.N., F^{15} 228^1).

74. A.N., F^{17} 2276, item 305, Carcassonne (Aude).

75. Ibid., item 319, Seurre-sur-Saône (Bellegarde), Côte-d'Or.

76. Ibid., item 316, Auch.

77. In the same sense, I find many expressions of the contempt and even of the hatred with which many surgeons pursued the matrons; yet I also notice an overlap between deliveries carried out by men (a "fashion" launched by Louis XIV) and by women. And finally, I note in the discourse of the enlightened physicians that marked the first empire the creation and justification of the "stereotype of femininity" analyzed by Yvonne Knibiehler in "Les Médecins et la nature féminine du temps du Code civil," *Annales, E.S.C.* 31 (July-August 1976): 824-45.

78. A.N., F^{17} 2276, item 294, Nuits, 29 December 1790. Unlike the men presented as sorcerers by our surgeons, no woman was called a "witch."

79. A.D. Gironde, C 3304, letter of 12 December 1786, signed by the priests of Castelnau and Avensac (Médoc).

80. Mandrou, *Magistrats et sorciers,* pp. 426 ff.

81. For their colleagues the parmacist-apothecaries, cf. Bénédicte Dehillerin, *"Le Collège royal de pharmacie de Paris, 1777-1795"* (Master's thesis, University of Paris-I, 1976).

82. J. Bernard, *Grandeur et tentation de la médecine* (Paris, 1973), p. 171.

83. S. Moscovici, *Essai sur l'histoire humaine de la nature* (Paris, 1968), p. 513, as well as the particularly enlightening conclusion. See also, on a different level of discourse, H. M. Koelbing, "Un Point de vue négligé par les médecins historiens: La Médecine de tous les jours," *Médecine et hygiène* 1 118, issues 9-10 (1974): 1-3.

2

Women, Religion, and Medicine

Jacques Léonard

The first Frenchwoman to receive a doctorate in medicine was granted her degree by the medical faculty of Paris in 1875.[1] But secondary education for girls progressed too slowly and prejudices remained too tenacious for a sizable tide of female medical students to follow this pioneer. It had not been a total victory. Women still had to win the right to compete for positions as externs (1881) and interns (1885). Even so, the first women physicians remained isolated within certain specific fields or in fields considered of secondary importance: female ailments, childhood diseases, and diseases of the eyes or skin.[2] This was a misogynous century, a society based upon male dominance. Our attention should focus upon this long ostracisim, which was also evident in public health departments and which in many respects was illogical. Although the law of 19 ventôse, year XI (10 March 1803), did not formally forbid women to practice medicine—and even granted midwives the major role in obstetrics—the antifeminist interpretations of this document soon became clear and removed any ambiguities about the interpretation of two statements made by legislators in 1803. One paragraph in the statement of the motives behind the law of 21 germinal, year XI (11 April 1803), concerning pharmaceutics explained why the old sufferance of pharmacists' widows who continued their husbands' businesses would have to cease: "You will note that since pharmacy is less a trade than a scholarly profession, it must consequently be closed to women." The "consequently" was peremptory, and women were *a fortiori* excluded from medicine. This was confirmed by Chaptal's circulating letter dated 13 fructidor, year XII (31 August 1803), which commented upon an article in the law of ventôse: "The exercise of the art by women, by empirics, by people exercising another trade, or at public spectacles, by men who are dishonored or censured by

Annales, E. S. C. 32 (September-Oct. 1977): 887-907. Translated by Patricia M. Ranum.

public opinion, can in no manner be authorized by the article in question."[3]
The list speaks for itself; the reason behind it is understood.

But this legal eviction of women was in actual fact untenable because it was basically paradoxical. Indeed, on all sides clergy, Rousseauists, romantics, and so forth, described in a favorable light female sensitivity (charity, benevolence, gentleness) and the virtues and aptitudes that gave women their place in the home, their role as mothers, and their natural and social vocation to care for loved ones, especially children and the aged. In rural France a woman was traditionally responsible for the water, the fire, the kitchen, the poultry yard, the stable, and sometimes the garden. These tasks show clearly that her role was to care for the animals and the health of the members of the household. For routine childbirth a *matrone* [a woman with no official training, but experienced in helping with deliveries] or a trained midwife was called in. Modesty and complicity placed certain intimate matters in the realm of the distaff. In short, actual fact won out over juridical principles, and the majority of women practiced medicine without a diploma, just as Monsieur Jourdain, in Molière's *Bourgeois Gentilhomme,* spoke prose [i.e., as a matter of course]. Still, some women assumed therapeutic responsibilities outside their families. Leaving aside the very interesting categories of midwife, *matrone,* charitable noblewoman or middle-class woman, witch, and healer, I shall examine the plentiful and varied troops of charitable sisters[4] and members of religious orders who cared for the sick jn hospitals, hospices, asylums, orphanages, and shelters, in urban dispensaries and relief offices, and in rural dispensaries.

How and why, after the Revolution of 1789, did women resume a major role in public health? What components shaped the quarrel between women and physicians? What direct or indirect contribution did women make to providing medical services for the common people?[5]

The Blossom Time of Nuns' White Headdresses

After the upheavals of the Revolution, from which religious houses suffered especially, the return of these religious congregations during the Consulate can be compared with that of the nobles who had emigrated during the troubles and with the pacification being worked out under the religious Concordat. Their return is a well-known aspect of the Restoration and went hand in hand with the progressive, social, educational, and political re-Catholicization. Those holding power were concerned with scholarship and patronage and, as we know, promoted activities on this intermediate level. But the impetus did not come totally from the top. Social clericalism was also meeting urgent needs that had arisen spontaneously among the people on the local level, needs that leading citizens and taxpayers were only too happy to meet at reduced cost.

It is easy to find justifications for the authorities' urgent calling back of the nuns. Châteaubriand was one of the foremost spokesmen and, in book 6 of the *Génie du Christianisme,* he listed the services rendered to society by the clergy, alluded to hospitals and nuns, and recalled the traditional gray-garbed sisters in rural areas:

How affecting was the sight of a young, beautiful, and compassionate female performing, in the name of God, the office [i.e., profession] of physician for the rustic! . . . They, as well as all their sisters, were remarkable for the neatness of their external appearance and a look of content indicating that body and soul were alike free from stain. They were full of tenderness, but yet were not deficient in firmness to endure the sight of human sufferings, and to enforce the obedience of their patients. They excelled in setting limbs broken by falls, or dislocated by those accidents so common in the country: but a circumstance of still greater importance was, that the Grey Nun never failed to drop a word concerning God in the ear of the husbandman, and that never did morality assume forms more divine, for the purpose of insinuating itself into the human heart.[6]

Nuns were, therefore, necessary if moral values were to be respected. In the hospitals for which lay nurses could not be recruited, the nuns provided the most economical and most reassuring solution. Thus Chaptal put them back to work in the hospitals as of 1 nivôse, year IX (22 January 1801). He encountered no legal difficulties on this score, but for diverse reasons some sisters of charity refused to "resume their former estate" and on occasion preferred to practice medicine illegally.[7]

How were these nuns able to expand the circle of their nursing activities beyond the hospital walls? The specific situations varied, but three imprudent texts encouraged them to become impromptu pharmacists. One was a directive from the Paris medical school, dated 9 pluviôse, year X (29 January 1802), applicable to hospices and to institutions providing care at home, which permitted nuns to prepare "teas, oily potions, simple potions, simple soothing emulsions to be sipped by patients, cataplasms, fomentations, medicines, and other similar magistral medications whose preparation is so simple that it requires no very extensive knowledge of pharmacology."[8] The other document, more official in nature, justified the zealousness of rural nuns. I am referring to the circular sent out by Champagny, minister of the interior, on 12 floréal, year XIII (2 May 1805). This circular followed the pattern of the charitable procedures customary curing the Ancien Régime and reorganized help for the poor during epidemics, recommending that the prefects [of the various French departments] "multiply as much as possible the number of sisters of charity in their departments and link them wherever means permit to charitable institutions for the poor." Another note, this time from Crétet, minister of the interior, dated 1 November 1806, brought complete reassurance for the nuns. They would not be affected by article 25 of the law of germinal (dealing with the practice of pharmacology) if the medications they distributed came from hospital pharmacies. But this was not always the case; indeed, far from it. During this first phase it was a question of helping the poor and not a matter of selling remedies.

After 1815 calls went out for great numbers of nuns, the priority being given to conservative regions: the France of the châteaux, the France of the Chouans and the royalists. If the ecclesiastical and legitimist authorities, and the leadership within the clergy, encouraged this massive induction of nuns, it was because these women made it possible to solve, cheaply and in accordance with the practices of the Ancien Régime, a few of the social problems in the provinces. Through charity and catechism, these leaders hoped simultaneously to end poverty and discontent and to separate the "true poor," the resigned and deserving poor, from the ungrateful individuals and outcasts. This required calling into question the vast and shifting category of those who needed help—a shifting category because chance economic circumstances were added to reasons having to do with the structure of society. Indeed, it is not enough to focus upon the needy, the eternal victims of extreme and permanent poverty, who apparently were the individuals most exposed to biological misfortune. We must not forget that the large majority of the nonindigent —small farmers, hired farm hands, workers in workshops and factories, artisans, clerks and office employees who had no family wealth, and even members of the middle class living off their income—might easily teeter and drag their families down into poverty when an accident, illness, or old age prevented them from working. Independent of periods of unemployment or epidemic, sizable numbers of people constantly were unable to free themselves from relative or absolute, temporary or permanent, financial difficulties, physical or mental weakness, or some other shortcoming. Alms or the poorhouse did not offer a satisfactory solution for people of this sort. Overwhelmed by discouragement, they had to be helped tactfully. The nuns brought them at one and the same time support for their soul, financial aid, and care for the body. This was the virtuous sphere of social clericalism that captivated Maistre and Bonald.

By the time of the Restoration the fruitful association between dispensary and school had been established. Rural townships supplied lodgings and a small allowance, the general councils of the various departments of France authorized an annual subsidy, and rich philanthropists ensured their salvation by increasing these sums through legacies. This made possible the creation of institutions in which teaching nuns, nurses who tended the sick at home, woman pharmacists, or hospital nurses lived together. But the pupils' parents contributed little money, and the upkeep of these small rural schools required other, more regular sources of income; hence the idea of selling medications prepared by these little dispensaries to rich or well-to-do families. According to good, charitable logic, the profit was officially supposed to go to improving the facilities of the dispensaries and thus to helping the poor. In reality, part of this income, which was more or less illegal,[9] went to the superiors of these religious congregations and supported elementary schools and workrooms for girls. As we shall see, such operations were quite profitable.

After 1830 [and the fall of the Restoration Monarchy] the nuns remained indispensable; the movement could only gain in strength. Indeed, in many regions, without the nuns how could the authorities have applied or attenuated the Guizot law of 1833, the Pelet de la Lozère law of 1836, and above all the Falloux law of 1850? Money was short. Taxpayers and their representatives balked; churches and manses in need of reconstruction competed with hospitals, schools, and roads. The choice had to be made. The leading citizens opted for the easiest course and preferred to give a little help to pious girls, who as a result could earn their own living. "Everywhere they are given preference by administrative and judicial authorities, in defiance of the law."[10] The medical convention held in November 1845 was wasting its time when it expressed the general desire that "hospitals, administrative establishments, charitable institutions, and other establishments of that sort cannot have a pharmacy on the premises for their daily needs unless the preparation of the medications is entrusted to a pharmacist, and *unless they are prevented from ever selling, retailing, or even distributing any medication beyond the premises.*" When, in June-July 1847, the Chamber of Peers debated Salvandy's medical reform, Montalembert successfully defended the sisters of charity.

During the Second Empire, in certain departments of the nation, plans were drawn up for free medical services for the poor in rural areas. It seemed quite advisable to include in this program both the nuns already on the spot and active and those, in some cases even more numerous, who had been mobilized by the application of the Falloux law. "The most practical and efficient means of attaining the proposed goal is to establish in the countryside sisters of charity who, independent of their devotion for suffering humanity, will provide an example of all the Christian virtues."[11] The General Council of the Breton department of Côtes-du-Nord therefore shared Chateaubriand's opinion. Departmental assemblies and great landowners provided the initial funds for these dispensaries, especially between 1855 and 1865. This alliance between political and social leaders was frequently denounced by physicians and by republicans. Dr. Chevandier, from the department of Drôme, who was representative of both groups, stated:

Extending its influence and increasing its wealth seems to be the clergy's two-pronged concern. Every mother house has control over the nun who cares for the children and the nun who cares for the sick. Since the parish priest helps, we can see what influence this trinity is acquiring by constant involvement in medicine, education, and religion. Medicine serves as a skeleton key for the other two, which take advantage of this to gain entry into families and to find students for their religious schools.[12]

However, the situation in Drôme was less all-encompassing than that in the department of Morbihan, as denounced by a physician at Auray: "The nuns are entrusted by the townships with caring for the poor. Under the direct suggestion of the large landholders, who are the political and religious allies of these merchant communities, the workers are expected to tolerate the exploiting woman pharmacist who intrudes at their bedsides. Those whom wealth makes independent find it easiest to go along with this scandalous system of charity."[13] In regions where clericalism was progressing openly, and/or during periods when it was undisguisedly expanding, nuns also participated in drawing up the lists of the town's indigents. Thus, they could select those who were eligible for charity and sell to the others, with impunity and in broad daylight, the remedies they dispensed along with medical advice. In the midst of the so-called anticlerical period, the president of the physicians' union of the department of Finistère displayed, with anguish and indignation, a plan for a parochial school in which the architect had allocated a space for "consultations and remedies."[14]

I doubtlessly should conclude this chronological bird's-eye view with a statistical table. It is not enough to report that in almost every part of France these illegal dispensaries were more numerous than certified pharmacies by the late 1860s. Take, for example, the Sisters of Wisdom in Brittany. They were active in three fields: orphanages, hospitals, and rural institutions for "instruction-charity-pharmacy." Table 2.1 shows the dates at which their various services were established in Brittany. The two decades following the Falloux law of 1850 appear to have been years of euphoria. In 1850 the Sisters of Wisdom were present in fifty-one Breton townships; in 1870, in eighty-one townships, for a 60 percent increase.[15] Now, there obviously were other nursing congregations, for which similar phenomena can be noted. In the diocese of Rennes, twenty-four new congregations were authorized between 1850 and 1860, compared with twenty-one between 1815 and 1850.[16]

Table 2.1—Services Established by the Sisters of Wisdom

Date	Orphanages	Hospitals	Rural
Before the Revolution	8	16	8
Consulate, Empire	3	6	1
Restoration	2	4	7
July Monarchy	3	0	6
1850-70	8	7	21
1870-79	2	1	7
After 1879 (till 1900)	2	3	3

The time has come for me to provide a more profound explanation for this success of the nuns and to shed some light on two powerful factors in any interpretation: the community of interest between the Catholic way of life and biological misfortune on the one hand, and the obvious collusion between women and nuns on the other. I am not trying to oversimplify the question. Other explanatory schemes could be proposed and preferred. My interpretation of these facts is inspired consciously—and perhaps even more so unconsciously—by a long period spent consulting archives relating to medicine and physicians.

Many Catholics spontaneously turned to religious practices in order to obtain a cure: they would pray, light a candle before the statue of a thaumaturgical saint, go on a pilgrimage, and so forth. Their conduct was legitimated by the Gospels themselves. I need not emphasize the multiple miraculous cures by Jesus, whose power was transmitted to the apostles: "Heal the sick,"[17] he said. "Then he called his twelve disciples together and gave them power

and authority over all devils, and to cure diseases."[18] The book of Acts
mentions both the individual healings by Peter and (especially) by Paul and
the mass cures. In addition, by the laying on of hands, the seventy-two
disciples and those who believed in the Gospel could cast out devils and work
miracles. Although the nineteenth-century faithful never or almost never read
the Scriptures, they had a direct and repeated acquaintance with them because
everything relating to the thaumaturgical merit of Jesus, the apostles, and the
saints served as an argument in favor of the truth of Catholicism and was
frequently evoked in the "propers of the day" and repeated with gusto in
Sunday sermons. Although the mass was in Latin, the congregation could
read the Gospel and the Epistle in French in their missals, and sermons
were given in French or, even better, in the local dialect. When dealing with
congregations composed of the common people, the clergy did not try to
interpret these miracles as healings of the soul, conversions of the heart, or
victories over sin; each priest limited himself to a literal and realistic interpretation. Indeed, this also encouraged the countless pious engravings and pictures
commemorating first communions that were printed by such publishers as
Alfred Mame of Tours. At the end of the nineteenth century, specialized
prayers, prayers for exorcisms, and guides for novenas were still in circulation.
Although they multiplied uncontrollably, these were not local superstitions
but accepted practices of the Roman Catholic Church. One example is the
prayer addressed to Saint Michael the Archangel, published by order of Pope
Leo XIII with a detailed explanation stating that "one will use it especially in
cases where one can presume an action by the devil, manifest in either the
wickedness of men or in temptations, illnesses, bad weather, and calamities of
all sorts."[19]

In general, numerous intercessors were mobilized in this way for therapeutic
ends; angels, guardian angels, prophets, martyrs, confessors, virgins, and above
all saints reputed to overcome illness were invoked. Now, in the nineteenth
century, during the years when ultramontanism was increasing, veneration of
the Virgin and related practices were also spreading, as evidenced in such
confraternities as the Sacred Heart, the Holy Sacrament, the Holy Rosary,
and so forth. And we know that the nuns zealously spread these pious
practices; they shared with rural women an extreme enthusiasm for such
pilgrimage sites as La Salette, Lourdes, and Pontmain.

The nuns' success with the common people stemmed from the fact that
they were part of both the Church and womanhood. Paragons of chastity,
they did not reveal secrets that were better kept hidden, as certain *matrones*
or midwives did, nor did they make insolent jests. They blessed fertile wombs,
and nothing more. Teachers or catechists, they shaped young girls' minds
and remained their advisers once they had become wives and mothers. They
knew which physician should be consulted and to which saint one should
address one's prayers. They were on the same wave length as the peasants.
The tight purse strings of the country woman are a commonplace; the old
parsimony based on the land combined with and strengthened solidarity

among women. The physician and the pharmacist often lived too far away. Going to fetch or notify the physician, waiting until he came and then paying someone to go to town if the physician was not also a propharmacist (that is, if he himself was not permitted to distribute the remedies he prescribed), in order to have the pharmacist fill the prescription, and then waiting again—all this took time. "You see what a waste of time it would be for our poor and even for our farmers if they were obliged to waste almost an entire day in order to buy a remedy for fifty centimes."[20] The mayor was right; but the mistresses of households also knew that a per-kilometer supplement could greatly increase the physician's fee for a house call. The nun supplied the medication at once, with careful explanations. So why call a licensed practitioner if you had confidence in this stopgap female doctor? Besides, no one would complain about it. If she succeeded in making the trouble go away, you slipped a piece of money into her hand and sang her praises; if she failed—she, who was closer to the good Lord and his saints than the learned man—it was because Providence had willed it so. In regions where houses were far apart, nuns made the rounds on specified days; people waited for them to come by. Those who were not indigent realized that the nuns would not refuse to see them and would leave no one untreated. The nuns' directions were obediently heeded, for obeying these venerable virgins already constituted an act of piety.

The Grumbling by the Men in White

We know pious physicians who have ended up as veritable anticlericalists as a result of the incessant encroachment by nuns or parish priests into the medical world, an encroachment that often is harmful to the sick person, that very often is harmful to the physician's reputation as a result of more or less explicit criticisms, and that sometimes manages to compromise the practitioner's material situation or make it untenable.[21]

This confession by Dr. Henri Bon, one of the pillars of the respectable Society of Saint Luke, Saint Cosmos, and Saint Damien, an association of Catholic physicians, leads us to the vast question of nineteenth-century anticlericalism. We surely cannot ignore the philosophical reasons behind the flamboyant anti-Catholicism of certain physicians and politicians, such as Dr. Georges Clemenceau, Dr. Alfred Naquet, or Dr. Emile Combes, rather outdated silhouettes that retreat into the past and sometimes are gradually engulfed in our lack of comprehension.[22] Anyone who wants to understand the dispute between the medical profession and the clergy does not lack documents on the medical side. As a general rule, the texts go on at greater length about conflicts than they do about agreements; but in this instance we must make allowances for professional prudence. A physician could not risk alienating himself from an important fraction of his clientele by statements or actions that were hostile to dominant beliefs; a conformist competitor would soon supplant him. This is why handbooks on medical ethics advised future physicians to be reticent and indulgent: "You ought to avoid offending the religious ideas and convictions of your clients. Respect their scapulars, medals, and even the bottle of holy water from Lourdes that you see beside the medicine you have prescribed."[23] So how, in view of these circumstances, could we expect to see anything other than the open struggles, the visible part of the iceberg?

I shall begin by describing the different types of quarrels that pitted the women in white headdresses against the men in white coats. First I must draw a distinction between the closed world of the hospitals and the open world of the countryside.

In the hospitals, the detailed rules and the dominance of the hospital directors left no room for dissension between these two categories of "employees," the sisters and the physicians (who in the nineteenth century suffered from their rather subaltern position as far as hospital regulations and management were concerned). Their competition for influence was first of all expressed in conflicting material concerns. During the first sixty years of the nineteenth century, when the majority of institutions were decrepit and dilapidated and too small and crowded, the nuns often diverted structures from their medical use. In one place they managed to have priority given to the restoration or construction of their convent and its chapel; in another they used as a chapel a room that the physician wanted for other purposes. Money was short, and the nuns were in charge of the numerous abandoned children, old people, and invalids who were being "supported" in hospices. Why not put them to work? Had that not been done in the past [in the general hospitals of the Ancien Régime]? The sale of handicrafts outside the hospice provided a considerable source of income; too bad if "free" workers protested! In this way, spacious rooms were taken away from the sick and were transformed into workshops and sewing rooms, to the physicians' great displeasure.[24] It even happened that very small rural hospitals would disappear for a time, having been converted into mere relief offices, flanked by dispensaries, from which pharmacist-nuns went out into the surrounding area.

Hospital pharmacies were another source of discord. In theory, the nuns running these pharmacies were under the supervision of a licensed pharmacist, but in actual practice this supervision was fictitious in small hospitals and hospices, and even more so in rural charity offices. Thus, it was the mother superior who did the bulk purchasing and tried to buy drugs cheaply, in order to make small profits for the hospital by preparing medication that was not reserved solely for the indigent but was sold in the region without prescriptions and sometimes without precautions. With even more bitterness and undoubtedly better grounds for their accusations, physicians criticized the nuns in rural areas for obtaining supplies at discount, using adulterated products, and selling dangerous and toxic substances.

But even more serious was the fact that, according to their critics, the nursing nuns took advantage of their moral authority, to the detriment of the physicians' authority and at the expense of the public good. This "despotism," which varied with the period and with local circumstances, presupposed the alleged complicity of those in power within the clergy or, at the very least, indulgent acceptance by Catholic opinion. The nuns were merely meshes in the net that surrounded them. Let us look at the touchiest points. The rules of certain congregations prevented them from caring for men with venereal diseases and sometimes even from treating skin ailments. Carrying these prohibitions to extremes and invoking moral reasons, the nuns and their supporters succeeded in excluding from their hospitals certain individuals whom they considered undesirable: unwed mothers, prostitutes, and women with venereal diseases, three particularly overlapping categories. These patients were relegated to lying-in rooms, beggars' prisons, or prison infirmaries. This is why, during the first two-thirds of the nineteenth century, instruction in obstetrics and gynecology was paralyzed or greatly hindered in provincial medical schools, which worked through hospital clinics. When lying-in hospitals and services providing care and instruction at last became imperative, the nuns were careful to draw a distinction, among the pregnant women, between licensed prostitutes and indigent women. Likewise, for a long time they refused to permit the simultaneous presence of midwifery students and medical students in their establishments. It was even harder for them to overcome their repugnance for women with "shameful" illnesses. All their virtuous objections stood firm against the arguments of the populationists and medicohygienists, who only managed to assert themselves according to moral principles.

Inside the hospices the physicians' authority was particularly weak, since the boarders were given no intense or methodical therapy. These hospices were residences for orphaned or abandoned children, old people, or the peaceful insane. The power of these males, these physicians, was particularly diminished in the wards occupied by mentally ill women, where the nuns saw to it that strict discipline was maintained. They even inflicted inadmissable punishment, were free in their use of the strait jacket, and repeatedly used odious or merely puerile harassments upon the patients. When dealing with the mentally disturbed, they did not always understand the ideas and methods of reforming alienists, whom they suspected of wanting to absolve the patients of their sins by accusing society or by invoking purely physiological ailments.

In these medical establishments the nuns wanted to create an orderly and regular daily routine that would edify souls, and they tried to impose this regime upon the "medicos," who did not always define "good behavior" in the same way the nuns did. This led to incidents, noisy scenes, and altercations in which could be heard, "Down with the Béguines!"* With unremitting zeal the nuns tried to see that devotional duties were completed by the entire personnel, including the nurses and the girls serving as nurses' aides, whose status seems

---

*Created in the Low countries during the twelfth century, the lay sisterhoods called the Béguines can still be found in such cities as Brussels and Bruges. The women devote themselves to a religious life but take no vows and can leave the group and marry. In nineteenth-century France the name was applied pejoratively to nursing sisters.—Trans.

to have been unenviable in every respect. The sisters did not tolerate just any newspaper in their stations, where they decorated the walls with crucifixes and pious statuettes adorned with consecrated palm fronds. Anti-Catholic physicians attacked the moral pressure that the nuns exerted upon children and old people especially, their discourses about Hell, and their exploitation of the distress occasioned by physical suffering and separation from the family. "In these gloomy havens for the suffering, they have established an intolerable dictatorship of bigotry. They know how to take advantage of the paroxysms of anguish or delirium."[25] Yet few physicians, including those who stigmatized the nuns, asked for the prompt and complete laicization of the hospitals. The campaign for this purpose, led by Dr. Alfred Naquet and Dr. Désiré Bourneville between 1865 and 1885, met with almost total failure.[26]

Before closing this file, I wish that I could provide the opinions of those witnesses most concerned: the hospitalized patients themselves. But the indigent, the sick, and the afflicted are always the mutes of history.

The virtual trial of the rural nuns, which was conducted chiefly by physicians and various public officials who found clerical power distasteful, focused upon five accusations: obscurantism, incompetence, imprudence and negligence, love of money, and the demedicalization of certain regions.

Obscurantism! The word had been uttered! Were these holy women indeed on the side of the Enlightenment, science, and progress? Certain well-meaning individuals doubted it. Let us listen to their arguments. The nuns were suspected of a guilty indulgence toward the fatalistic form of providentialism: illnesses or accidents could be interpreted as punishments for a sin—an original sin, a mortal sin, or a long series of sins.[27] Suffering and even the mortification of the flesh assumed a positive value, serving to win the salvation of the soul. The nuns tended to sanction the biological resignation of lower-class women (and other women as well), their submissiveness toward repeated pregnancies, their more or less apathetic acceptance of the deaths of numerous very young children,[28] and the secrecy, the famous secrecy, within which sexual difficulties had to be cloaked, through modesty, shame, or obsession with sin.[29] Teachers of young girls, yet incapable of preparing them for their future roles as wives and mothers other than through the most automatic sort of conformity, the nuns taught the catechism while teaching the girls how to sew and sometimes gave the girls lessons in hygiene that ran counter to those being proclaimed by scientific physicians.[30] In general, they accepted or encouraged extramedical therapeutic measures, such as the veneration of healing saints; recourse to prayer, novenas, or pilgrimages; and hopes for miraculous cures. In the context of the day, a contrary position would have been inconceivable. And it would have been just as unconceivable for anticlerical physicians to denounce imprudent and shocking popular practices. For example, during widespread epidemics, physicians could scarcely prevent certain public assemblies of an expiatory and propitiatory nature—processions, public invocations, kissing the paten—that threatened to spread the contagion. They also became indignant over the custom of baptizing infants almost immediately after birth, undressing the child in the process, even during the winter months when the church was icy cold. What could they say about the hysterotomies carried out upon the bodies of pregnant women immediately after death in order to baptize the fetus, "a barbarous custom," in which nuns and ecclesiastics were involved![31]

Obscurantism, also, if they doubted scientific conquests. This question was posed early in the nineteenth century on the matter of the efficacy of smallpox vaccinations. "The nuns in this respect take a very difficult position, I might even say that their conduct is very reprehensible," scolded one of Napoleon's ministers in 1813.[32] Indeed, the nuns often could not or would not act counter to popular prejudices. When, during the 1860s, several departments as an economy measure gave up paying those who vaccinated poor children and put their trust in the good will of the local charitable services, the nuns running such services showed no great hurry. Quite the opposite. So the high mortality rates of 1870-71 are understandable. During the last quarter of the nineteenth century the nuns flouted the laws of the French Republic, admitting unvaccinated children into their schools and brazenly boycotting the measures against epidemics laid down by the authorities. Vaccination was not the only item questioned. According to their ages and regions, the nuns demonstrated more or less persistent and deep-rooted reticence about the rectal thermometer, subcutaneous injections, and chloroform during childbirth. Thus, to the dazzled eyes of the positivists, the exacerbated irrationalism of the nuns played a role in the history of human suffering that was sometimes sinister and sometimes ridiculous.

The second grievance against rural nuns was *incompetence*. It could be excused as involuntary, but it occupied a considerable place on the list. "Ignorant," "unlettered," "devoid of any form of instruction," "lacking all medical knowledge"—such were the insistent and redundant judgments expressed on all sides by physicians in charge of epidemics, members of medical examining boards or hygiene committees, professors in medical schools or faculties, pharmacists, mayors, subprefects, prefects, and magistrates. The superior of the Daughters of Wisdom must have been perfectly aware of this situation when he wrote them in 1867: "Avoid caring on your own for those serious and difficult ailments whose treatment requires studies you have not done and knowledge you have not acquired."[33] But didn't rural nuns receive their medical training in hospitals, under the supervision of physicians? Indeed, this sometimes was the case, but on the one hand congregations working in the countryside were not always represented in the hospitals and on the other the opposite procedure seems to have been more common. Young nuns, capable of bearing the fatigue involved in providing rural medical care, proved themselves in the country before being rewarded with relatively less arduous work in a hospital. In general, if a trio of holy women came to a village, the two most educated would run the tiny pharmacy and the school, and the most ignorant of the three—or the youngest—would go out into the neighborhood to care for the poor.

Imprudence and negligence were born of incompetence. According to my documentation, which is clearly promedical, the nuns in rural areas did not always take all the desirable precautions when storing, preparing, and distributing the remedies supplied by their dispensaries. They were accused of "the most deadly scorn" for dosages, especially in the case of toxic substances.[34] Some did not hesitate to use the knife, and thus a certain number would unwaveringly cut out tumors. Others—or perhaps the same ones—were ready to try the most daring measures and were obsessed with the lancet. After having bled a patient excessively, they did not dare call in a doctor, who would realize the extent of the error they had committed.[35] As long as licensed physicians could not pride themselves on major therapeutic successes, denunciations of incidents of this sort necessitated some degree of discretion. Then, during the 1860s, the various chapters of the general association of physicians of France began to draw up frightening lists of the crude, often tragic blunders of which their rivals were said to have been guilty. The tragic events were revealed. Finally, when these blunders became transformed into catastrophes such as measles or diphtheria epidemics from which the nuns had excluded the physicians, the tone became more strident, for the prestige so recently acquired by medical science henceforth made these marginal and dangerous activities intolerable. "One is led to the inexorable conclusion that instead of constituting a good for society, all these nuns on the contrary pose a real and permanent danger for it."[36]

The fourth reproach, *love of money,* addressed to rural nuns seems less dramatic. True, this economic grievance prompted a great deal of bitter writings. Like the pharmacist-nuns in the small hospices, whom I described earlier, those in rural dispensaries cheaply bought drugs of inferior quality sent to them by unscrupulous wholesalers or supplied by swarms of peddlers and traveling salesmen. Were they the victims or the accomplices? The question was a subject of debate, since the inspectors of pharmacies and other related shops wanted to have a clear conscience. So inspection visits would have to be permitted and would involve careful scrutiny. Yet, despite the law, many mayors, subprefects, and prefects did not want these inspections to reveal officially that these venerable women stocked secret remedies and toxic products, or that they prepared complex medications without prescriptions—infractions that would result in the closing of their dispensaries in persuance of the law. But the scandal spread. I have already explained why they sold as many medications as possible to well-to-do families, from whom they could ask good prices. Running their own shops, they "exploited" every social class, "taking to the rich man the numerous and varied potions that he is able to pay for, and sending to the poor man a banal and watered-down herb tea."[37] By making people pay for drugs only, the nuns permitted them to save the cost of the physician's fee and, therefore, in the world of artisans and peasants, constituted irresistible rivals of the medical profession.

This brings us to the final complaint, which threatened the positions of physicians and of future physicians and the medical services provided for the upper classes. It is true that this *demedicalization* was only seriously evident in those regions most under the clergy's sway. There the nuns aroused anxiety in middle-class families by driving out established physicians. Entire cantons, and sometimes adjoining cantons, lost their practitioners, in this way hastening the influx of other congreganists.* The extreme case was that of the department of Morbihan, where the number of physicians fell from 106 in 1841 to 67 in 1881, and where there were 89 illegal dispensaries managed by nuns in 1861 and 166 in 1884. In the western part of the Breton peninsula, the number of physicians per inhabitant declined as the number of pharmacist-nuns increased. The physicians involved were fully aware of this. One can imagine their bitterness toward "this tendency unceasingly shown by the clergy to gain control of the lucrative employment in our society."[38] Some even made more politically oriented judgments and denounced the bad organization of "public health": "Do not these charitable undertakings (which, moreover, constitute the illegal practice of medicine) prove that there is a lacuna in our benevolent institutions? As we see it, the guilty parties are those who tolerate a state of affairs that they are unwilling to change by giving the impoverished rural sick the physicians and medications necessary for their treatment."[39] These grumblings by the men in white permit us to measure the limits of their power during the nineteenth century. Two medical offensives against these stated abuses aborted, first during the Second Empire, which kept its distance from the Roman Catholic Church, and again during the 1880s, during the opportunistic anticlerical period.

To a large degree this struggle against the illegal practice of medicine cemented together the members of the medical profession. It is impossible to believe otherwise when one looks closely at the creation of the first Association Générale de Prévoyance et de Secours Mutuel des Médecins de France [general association for reserve funds and mutual help of the physicians of France], founded in 1858. This group began discreet or detailed inquiries locally, then moved on to polite overtures to the religious authorities, while their directors in Paris on the general council of the general association of French physicians tried to influence the government ministers concerned, and especially the minister for public education and religion. These physicians usually received favorable replies. Bishops drew up circular letters to warn the nuns, asking them to remember that they were prohibited from preparing medications in their dispensaries, selling any remedy whatsoever, and performing surgery. They were to note that, when watching with the sick, they were supposed to obey the principles of prudence and gratuitousness. But the nuns turned a deaf ear, knowing that they could always hide behind the excuse of an emergency when treating sick or injured peasants. "Charity is

---

*Congreganists: members of a congregation of laymen or laywomen who worked under the direction of ecclesiastics, frequently in schools or hospitals.—Trans.

ingenious, my dear sisters, I do not doubt that the fine virtue whose name you bear [i.e., the Sisters of Charity] inspires in you the ways by which to ease humanity's suffering."[40] Under such conditions, the dissuasive effect of the letters was minimal. Would the nuns have to be taken to court? The physicians encountered ironic or submissive judges who were always ready to be convinced that the nuns were providing their services gratis or who at best agreed to advise them to be more prudent. For the physicians, going before the courts meant risking being faced by intimidated, frightened, or hostile witnesses or by judges who believed they would be doing wrong in criticizing, even to a limited degree, these "holy women." Merely threatening to take nuns to court brought censure. Showing pious irritation, the sisters needed only to threaten to stop providing care, and petitions would circulate, leading citizens would warn the people to beware of physicians, the poor would assemble, and insults would rain down.

When the Third Republic—the republic of true republicans—was established, medical opinion, buoyed up by scientific success that was conferring honor and value upon "free" thought, counted on taking revenge. In actual fact, anticlerical politicians limited themselves to restricting the nuns' importance through a few minimal legal steps. For example, the visits to their dispensaries by pharmacy inspectors, specified by the law, henceforth were obligatory. Or else the mayors were obliged to select "from among individuals possessing diplomas"[41] those who were to vaccinate poor children, which theoretically would exclude the nuns. On the whole, and as far as the essential problem was concerned, despite official inquiries that forced the minister of justice, Jules Cazot, to admit "the seriousness of the facts," the authorities of the Third Republic showed maximum toleration. They surely did not want to rub salt into the open wound of the education question. Governing meant also knowing how to assess the importance of the facts, even disagreeable facts. Like the nursing nuns, these illegal pharmacist-nuns had become indispensible. The evil had been done; they could not be immediately replaced by registered nurses. The government could not "abruptly deprive of all pharmaceutical help certain rural populations who benefit from them."[42] The very recently created medical associations[43] tried to disregard this timidity shown by officialdom. Disappointed by the demurs of the ministers, they alerted the attorneys; but the courts, though warned, scarcely budged. These medical associations encountered the same stumbling blocks as the groups earlier created for "mutual help." The Republic demonstrated its indulgence clearly through the much-discussed article 16 of the law of 30 November 1892, which reorganized the medical profession. Indeed, in order to be affected by the sanctions punishing the illegal practice of medicine, the unlicensed individual would have to participate *"habitually, or by regular intent,* in the treatment of ailments or surgical affections, or the practice of the dental art or lying-in, *except in the case of an authenticated emergency."* The words I have italicized provided the nuns with an escape.

Furthermore, over the years they became more and more effective at adapting themselves to the gradual changes resulting from an increasingly efficient medical science, which, it must be admitted, they henceforth served remarkably well. The harshest criticisms collapsed of their own accord.

The Condominium

So war did not break out between the white headdresses and the white coats. I shall not try here to refute all the accusations that the physicians accumulated against the nursing nuns over the course of the nineteenth century, but a closer reading of the records will reveal the deep-seated reasons for the de facto compromise made by the two groups. We know that society will tolerate contradictions for a long time if they are advantageous. The century of romanticism and scientism ran its entire course in a state of permanent disequilibrium; the pros and the cons dealt fairly with one another.

On a closer look we see that, although they were the trustees of the most venerable traditions, the nuns never really put themselves in a position where they would oppose "scientific" medicine. They were by no means the agents of a magical antimedicine, or a feminine counterpower, or a peasant counter-culture. With few exceptions, they were not witches. True, in their hands medicine and official pharmacies were more or less consciously pushed aside, glossed over, as local customs and resources dictated. Here and there the nuns annexed any old wives' recipes that seemed worthwhile, innocently incorporated a few paganizing or christianized rituals, and made a great use of the animals and produce of the farm and the fruits and vegetables of the garden. Far from the city, they improvised, taking liberties with the *Codex* [of pharmaceutical formulae] as well as with the law of ventôse. This was medicine, tempered by distance; but there was no difference between the nature of their medicine and that practiced by physicians. The proof is that the nuns had medical kits; they used the physicians' or surgeons' implements (cupping glasses, lancets, scalpels); they bled and purged, imposed fasts, or administered quinine. They imitated medical prescriptions, to the degree that it was possible. Sometimes they had access to the entire gamut of phar-macopoeia, buying their drugs in bulk from pharmacists and later, as soon as they appeared, enthusiastically adopting ready-prepared specialties in pill form. On their level they were already introducing medicine and pharma-cology, under the banners of charity, to people who sometimes refused to accept those "sciences."

Here we must return to the question of how much medical information these nuns possessed in order to see the nuances behind the criticism of their being intellectually void that hovers over certain documents. Books such as the *Manuel de médecine et chirurgie à l'usage des soeurs hospitalières* [medical and sugical handbook for the use of nursing nuns] (Nantes, 1836) were written for their use. Sister Philomène, in the novel by that name written by the Goncourt brothers in 1861, was studying "a bit of basic medicine." In

the hospitals the nuns were advised to keep their eyes and ears open during
the rounds of the chief physicians. During such sessions they learned whatever
these physicians deigned to teach them. The results, therefore, depended in
part upon the patience and teaching ability of the physicians on the hospital
staff. Aided by experience, some nuns ended up knowing more than a public
health officer. Sometimes, with their smattering of Latin, they felt less at a loss
than others in pharmacology. It was said that rural nuns were not "lettered,"
that they had no knowledge of rhetoric and grammar; but they were rarely
illiterate. Physicians (medical students, journalists, or professors) wrote
numerous books and periodicals, thus disseminating medical information via
peddlers and other means. These works bear evocative titles: *Manuel de
santé* [Health handbook], *Vrai Manuel de la médecine des pauvres* [True
handbook on medicine for the poor], *Avis au peuple sur sa santé* [Notice to
commonfolk on their health], *Conseils aux mères* [Advice for mothers], *La
Santé pour tous* [Everyone's health]. The subtitles are no less eloquent. They
were addressed to the leading citizens, the residents of châteaux, the mistresses
of households, and, naturally, the nuns. One book encouraged the practice of
self-medication; another claimed to be the "guide for mothers and nurses to
curing the illnesses of their children."[44] Some authors specialized in matters of
hygiene and wanted to influence the lay public. One prospectus for a "serious"
medical journal recommended that it be read by "mayors, parish priests,
landlords, heads of business, mothers, and charitable ladies"[45] and shows not
the least trace of jealous protection of a professional monopoly. Indeed, it
accepted the risk that it would contribute to facilitating the illegal practice of
medicine. Why would the nuns who cared for the sick not have access to this
useful and varied literature? They also had at their disposal certain administrative documents concerning first aid for the drowning and asphyxiated,
mushroom poisoning, bites by rabid animals, snake bites, and so forth—all of
which could be considered "emergencies," in view of the geographical dis-
tances separating the patients from medical help.

The nuns' educational levels and their concern with medical information
depended to a large degree on their social origins. Therefore, a statistical
study should be made of the families of these nursing nuns. Although the
majority seem indeed to have been local girls from rural families, in the west
of Brittany it can be observed, though no exact tally has been made, that
physicians often had daughters, sisters, or cousins in nursing orders. In passing,
I should like to describe briefly this social milieu. Education for the sons of
the family was very costly and made it difficult to provide a suitable dowry for
the daughters. Hence, a large proportion of these girls remained unmarried.
Those who wanted to devote their lives to others and who could not study
medicine entered a religious order or a third order. They were all the more
eager to do so because, by devoting themselves to suffering humanity, they
were, in nun's garb, imitating the vocation or profession of a father or brother
whom they admired and were also making the most of a certain vague
experience with medicine learned in their family circle. But the religious

conviction of a Catholic also had to enter into this choice! Now, these combined circumstances occurred within veritable dynasties of clericalist and royalist physicians, physicians serving châteaux, convents, and rectories. These were the same families that, in addition, gave birth to priests, papal zouaves,* and conservative politicians. And from them came the nuns who climbed to positions of responsibility and who, as "mothers superior," for example, provided an emotional and cultural link between clerical power and medical power.

Extending beyond polite conversation, this link was expressed in a veritable professional alliance with undeniable psychological impact. Physicians frequently concealed the nuns' illegal practice of pharmacology and emergency medicine and worked with them in a productive manner. If the nuns were accused or harassed, the physicians loudly declared that these women were carrying out their orders, and that ended that. They supported or, if need be, patched up the nun's doings. When widespread epidemics broke out, after first having made the rounds in the region themselves, the physicians ceded to the nuns their right to treat the sick. And they expressed their satisfaction that the sisters were there to see that their orders were being carried out locally. In the minds of many doctors, it was sufficient to supervise the nursing activities of the nuns, as the physician in the Ancien Régime had supervised the minor surgeons and as the new sort of doctor in certain cases was still obliged to look over the shoulders of midwives with second-class diplomas or health officers. Only too happy not to be obliged to waste time traveling over rutted roads or making poorly paid visits to change smelly dressings, these physicians preferred to have the nuns continue to filter calls so that the poor could not make excessive demands upon the medical profession.

Here we are far from the rigid claims made by anticlerical factions that the nuns showed a traditionalist obscurantism. On the contrary, as if exchanging good for good, when a practitioner was needed, the nuns called in the one they preferred, that is, the one who thought as they did. Through their interpersonal relationships, they kept rival physicians whom they would be unwilling to recommend from settling in the area or prevented the arrival of a pharmacist who would take from the "good" local doctor the right to be a pharmacist, that is, the right to deliver medications to his own clients.[46] They influenced well-to-do families, selected from among the licensed physicians those who demonstrated the best moral principles, and arbitrated to the advantage of those who had a pew reserved in the local parish churches, constituting an exclusive claque in their favor. One mayor candidly recognized that "the physician who is habitually consulted by our sick folk openly proclaims that he never had so many clients until the nuns arrived."[47] The nuns had no difficulty in identifying physicians faithful to the Church: for example, those who would hasten to have a priest summoned to the bedside of someone

---

*Members of a special corps created in 1860 by General Lamoricière to defend the Papal State. Most zouaves were volunteers and came from the leading families of France. — Trans.

who might be dying. At times the interests of clergy and physicians seem to have been intermeshed. The clergy—which played a leading role in marriages, inheritances, clienteles, education, good jobs, and the "top posts" of the medical bourgeoisie,[48] and which provided confessors and teachers in "free," that is, parochial, schools—enjoyed providing information to the nursing nuns. Strong networks of former students of the various religious secondary schools existed in such organizations as the Good Deeds, the Good Books, the Good Press, the Society of Saint Vincent de Paul, lay congregations, patronage groups for apprentices, and church vestries. These networks formed chains of solidarity and provided places in which to meet. Nor should we forget the founding of the Catholic faculty at Lille in 1887, the Conférence Laennec in 1879, and the medical society of Saint Luke, Saint Cosmos, and Saint Damien in 1884 (which brought together those physicians who were members of the clergy); or the pilgrimages to Rome, Saint-Anne-d'Auray, and above all Lourdes organized by nuns and Catholic physicians.

In all events, the nuns brought physicians into the homes of the humble families with whom they were acquainted. They introduced the faithful to medicine, at times combating the fatalistic attitudes of this rural population. They accustomed the people to view calling the doctor as a normal and, soon, an indispensible step. The nun's very attitude conferred worth upon the "good doctor," the "great doctor." "The doctor said that, . . ." "The doctor wants you to . . ."—such little phrases had the same ring as "Monsieur the Priest said that. . . ." Zealous and respectful, they inspired families to mimic this deference and submission. In this way they demonstrated and spread the significance of man, of science, and of the man of science. Hence the eager cooperation shown by countless physicians who took advantage of this marvelous publicity, this shift of power from the clerical to the medical and —closely copying the nuns—infiltrated everywhere.

Despite the disputes that arose, physicians approved of close cooperation with nursing nuns at patients' bedsides, at both ends of the spectrum: the most repugnant tasks of caring for the physical body (including washing cadavers and wrapping them in their shrouds) and the more spiritual troubles of the soul (anguish).

The first of these two functions was commonplace. On the one hand, the nuns tended to replace the minor surgeons who, during the Ancien Régime, had carried out the tasks—purgings, bleedings, dressings—prescribed by those entitled to wear the square-shaped hat of the physician. In addition, they did what the physician, who was not on the spot or who was in a hurry, could not or did not want to do. He merely stopped by; they returned to do the dirty work and linger over unsightly wounds. In this instance the hyperbole found in the praises sung of such nuns is easy to understand: "Angels of charity, devotion, and gentleness," willingly assumed humility, a Christian example.

At the other end of the spectrum of human troubles, physicians were not always displeased with the psychological impact of the nuns' conversations. They had to admit that certain sick people could be helped by other things than medicine. Dr. Henri Liégard concluded his thesis on the healing saints on a conciliatory note: "As a physician, I keep in mind that when our remedies prove powerless, one fortunately can still turn to religion."[49] These unusual possibilities must not be neglected, as one anticlerical doctor noted, grumblingly:

It is even profitable for the physician to take advantage of the unconscious suggestive state of his client for therapeutic ends and to urge him on to the miracle, if he is one of those who believes in miracles. I was an intern in a hospital ward in which there was an intelligent nun who, when she was preparing the sick to leave for Lourdes, would ask us whether such and such a patient would profit from his journey. Thanks to her fortunate initiative, we spared the incurable the fatigue of a long journey and perhaps favored the healing of purely functional symptoms in nervous patients.[50]

And, when meaning had to be given to the ultimate suffering, when the hour of death had come, the physician would tiptoe out and cede his place to the nun.

Even more frequently, nuns had to serve as intermediaries between the physicians' cold terminology and anxious families, who wanted a translation of sorts. The sisters leapt social and verbal barriers because they could talk to women. Female complicity and chatter established a certain sociability, especially in the countryside or in small towns. Compassionate and helpful, the nuns polarized the favor and even the fervor of the women. Mediators between the intellectual bourgeoisie and the weaker sex, they announced good and bad news and handed out minor secrets and topical advice. This was the meat and potatoes of their social task.

If there was one realm where their role *could* expand, it was in hygiene. For example, baths, which often were opposed on moral grounds, were only accepted if the nuns insisted. Fumigation by acids as developed by Guyton de Moreau [1737-1816] and disinfection with chlorides in private homes often depended upon the nuns' intervention. They could speak to the rural people and dissuade them from washing their laundry or vegetables in watering troughs or retting ponds. Their opinion was decisive as far as the cleanliness or feeding of infants was concerned; they had the right to decide the life or death of the population of bedbugs and lice. After the discovery of microbes, their zealousness was needed for another mission: convincing lower-class women of the need to fight this modern embodiment of Evil; convincing them to incorporate into household traditions the need to be clean, to teach children to wash their hands, to see that water or milk was boiled, to use abundant chlorine bleach, to burn the belongings of people with contagious illnesses, and so forth—all procedures that shared the prestige in which the new science basked. Young physicians and young nuns trod side by side along the carbolic acid paths to antisepsis and asepsis. Disinfecting ovens, autoclaves, sterile gloves and implements, immaculate white coats—all of this pleased the nuns' love of detail. Vaccinated against doubt by their profound conformism, they appreciated and enthusiastically spread the certitudes of bacteriological medicine, once those certitudes had been approved by the academics at the top of the medical pyramid.

We all know that smallpox vaccinations won acceptance by the public only to the degree that the clergy approved them publicly. During the First Empire, prefects requested that the bishops have the priests announce the rounds of vaccinating physicians, but not always with success. In short, "Outside the Church, no vaccinations." During the first three decades of the nineteenth century, the nuns had to be persuaded to vaccinate the orphans in a hospice or the children in a shelter. "As long as the clergy does not consider it a duty to announce vaccinations, we can be certain that this procedure will not spread far beyond the somewhat educated class," noted a disappointed prefect in 1818.[51] If the Church would stop viewing smallpox as a divine punishment, nothing would prevent it from rallying to the cause of prevention: "Vaccination is a protection that Providence has permitted us to discover and that we should consider among its blessings."[52] The flexibility of providentialism lubricates any reversals of position.

While on the subject of smallpox, let us go back to the days of calamitous epidemics, when the network of rural dispensaries served as the logistical base for distributing help. The physicians generally blamed malnutrition and poverty, which clearly were factors in the terrible epidemics of dysentery during the summer and fall months, and proposed to the authorities that clothing, blankets, linens, soups, bread, and sometimes meat and wine be made ready and distributed. Assisted by charitable individuals, the nuns carried out these plans, as they traditionally had. And thus, another web of medical-clerical complicity was woven from village to village. There was one objection to be skirted: certain specialists in contagious diseases complained about the nuns' heroic lack of caution when caring for smallpox or cholera victims. This daring was chiefly explained by their faith: "We pray to the good Lord," they would cheerfully say, "and we accept death if He wishes it."[53] But we must not forget that in their writings many physicians—the majority and the elite—long supported the theory blaming infection rather than contagion (especially in the cases of cholera and dysentery) and refused to alarm the population. On the contrary, they wanted to galvanize the family and social solidarities that certain nuns were carrying to the point of a mystical incandescence.

Another very striking issue is the way in which colonization overseas brought nuns and physicians together. Although anticlerical feelings among army and navy doctors persisted, nuns and physicians helped one another, despite a few hitches. They formed a brotherhood of Europeans, spread the use of vaccination, cared for eyes that were covered with flies, distributed quinine, and simultaneously spread the French language and advice about cleanliness. The physicians were pleased to see the nuns teaching reading, writing, and the catechism and enabling the inhabitants to understand and appreciate the doctors' orders. The nuns were happy to see that Western, Christian civilization was proving technically superior to that of the natives: healing also mean convincing, in other words, converting. And so, in the colonies, physicians and nuns became accustomed to helping one another, an experience that neither group would forget.[54]

The question sometimes is asked: How did the "Enlightenment" trickle down to the people? The process I have just described is a typical illustration of how this worked during the nineteenth century. In sum, like the Catholic physicians, the nuns finally surrendered to science. The sick person no longer was essentially the victim of human sins and divine punishment, but the victim of his milieu and his heredity. The theology of second causes easily confirmed this: although the first cause was omnipotent and unknowable, medicine and the other sciences revealed second causes in respect to which the experimental and rational spirit could function freely.

More specifically, despite a few failures, in many regions the white headdress and the white coat often worked quite well together. In any event, we can see no strict opposition between clerical and medical power. The nuns occupied a strategic position at the intersection of these two domains, domains with blurred frontiers. Although they transmitted the ideology of resignation and could thus be classed on the side of those who refused medicine, they were also militants on the side of the ideology of charity, which mobilized them as enthusiastic supporters of medicalization.

Everyone knows that the medical world is not an unfissured monolith—far from it. At the same time, during the nineteenth century the clerical edifice began to show cracks, under the rough jabs of Promethean thought. There were physicians who preached on both sides of the fence, as did the nursing nuns themselves. As long as economic and social circumstances did not permit financing medical care for the poor in any other manner, public assistance sanctimoniously continued to espouse the charitable tradition. Sheltered by this continuity, medical procedures evolved rapidly. The ambivalence of the nuns, who were entrusted with multiple missions, made the transition easier. And later they innocently contributed to "clericalizing" medicine's role by conferring upon it the solemn prestige that the medical profession may be on the brink of losing during the final quarter of the twentieth century.

NOTES

1. Cf. Mme. Jacques Bertillon (née Caroline Schultze, Pole), "La Femme-médecin au XIXe siècle" (medical dissertation, Paris, 1888).

2. Jules Simon and Dr. Gustave Simon, *La Femme au XXe siècle* (1892), pp. 93-104.

3. To protect the interests of pharmacists' families, a decision of 25 thermidor, year XI, authorized widows nonetheless to keep their husbands' dispensaries open for a year, on condition that they were assisted by a capable and serious "student." Here again the woman was placed in a dependent position, despite her rights as owner. This subordinate position is clearly evident in the case of midwives. A physician had to supervise the training courses in childbirth for students preparing to be second-class midwives; physicians sat upon the panels

created to admit them; in the event of a difficult labor, midwives had to summon a doctor. In the case of dentistry, which was not a legal monopoly, the highest court of appeals agreed that even a woman could practice that art, "reduced to its material acts," since no diploma was involved (decrees of 23 February 1827 and 15 May 1846).

4. Attention is called to the tertiaries (who, strictly speaking, are called *bonnes soeurs*) in Claude Langlois, "Les Tiers Ordres du diocèse de Vannes," *Structures religieuses et célibat féminin* (1972).

5. For lack of space in this article I will provide only the references and not the quotations. My presentation is inspired by the documents I consulted in preparing my dissertation for the *doctorat d'Etat*, "Les Médecins de l'Ouest au XIXe siècle," to which I refer the reader (defended on 10 January 1976 at the University of Paris-IV).

6. François-René de Chateaubriand, *Oeuvres complètes*, ed. Pourrat (1836), 17: 14. English translation: *The Beauties of Christianity*, trans. Frederic Shobert (Philadelphia, 1815), p. 460.

7. Report of the medical panel for Mayenne in 1804, Archives nationales, Paris, F 17, 2425.

8. In theory, simple drugs were obtained from a known and competent druggist and the medications were dispensed by a licensed pharmacist. It goes without saying that physicians were the only ones qualified to prescribe these remedies. But how could they effectively check on the care given by the nuns in the home?

9. A circulating letter signed by Martignac, 16 April 1828, permitted nuns to sell certain remedies, which conflicted with a decree by the court of Bordeaux dated 28 January 1830 and which general orders issued on 31 January 1840 vainly sought to outlaw.

10. Dr. A. Toulmouche, Report to the society for the sciences and the arts of Rennes, 13 February 1839, in Archives départementales [hereafter cited as A.D.], Ille-et-Vilaine, 18 Td 1.

11. Resolution by the General Council of the department of Côtes-du-Nord, 2 August 1854.

12. *Le Concours médical* (1883), p. 634.

13. Report by Dr. Eonnet, dated 25 April 1883.

14. Report by Dr. Jules Maréchal, dated 19 July 1884. *Le Concours médical* (1884), p. 542.

15. Archives of the Provincial House of Rennes.

16. Information supplied by M. Lagrée; data provided to the general direction of religious cults in 1891.

17. Matt. 10: 8.

18. Luke 9: 1.

19. A prayer distributed by the abbey of Mont-Saint-Michel and reprinted by the bishop of Coutances and Avranches on 5 March 1955.

20. Letter from the mayor of a village in Mayenne, dated 20 June 1890 (A.D., Mayenne, M 1452).

21. Dr. Henri Bon, *Précis de médecine catholique* (1935), p. 580.

22. Victor Hugo had a Bernardine nun say, "A physician: *that* believes in nothing" (*Les Misérables*, ed. Nelson, 2: 193).

23. Dr. Etienne Martin, *Précis de déontologie . . .* (1914), pp. 55-56.

24. They often did basketwork, spinning, weaving, or sewing. Minister Duchâtel criticized the "spirit of speculation" motivating the nuns in his circular dated 31 January 1840 (chap. 8, art. 39).

25. Dr. Ernest Coerderoy, anarchist physician, *Pour la Révolution: Jours d'exil* (1885; reprint ed. 1972), p. 192.

26. Bourneville was the promotor of lay nursing schools, for which he wrote the course handbooks.

27. Indeed, the Church upheld the thesis that sin had a pathogenic action (Bon, *Précis de médecine*, pp. 3, 392-408).

28. When a child died, people would repeat the proverb, "What God has given, God has taken away." And the sisters of charity used to say that a baptised child who died became "an angel of the good Lord" (letter by Dr. Angebault, dated 26 March 1840, A.D., Loire-Atlantique, 1 M 1358).

29. "Rural people view all ailments of the genitals as shameful and prefer to suffer greatly and even risk death rather than make them known" (letter from Perrigault, a public health officer, 1830, A.D., Loire-Atlantique, 1 M 1355).

30. In one Breton village, where a little girl had died of diphtheria, a schoolteacher-nun brought three pupils to kiss their classmate's face piously. Infected, two of these little girls

died (Dr. Gascon, of Redon, report dated 9 April 1885, A.D., Ille-et-Vilaine, 20 Mg 7).

31. Report by the *procureur général* on a custom in the arrondissement of Montfort, dated 22 August 1837 (A.D., Ille-et-Vilaine, 20 Mr 4). See also the incident at Abondance, in Haute-Savoie, reported in *Le Concours médical* (1883), p. 140, and in *Le Voltaire*, 22 May 1882.

32. Letter from Montalivet, minister of the interior, to Barante, prefect of the department of Loire-Inférieure, dated 6 November 1813 (A.D., Loire-Atlantique, 1 M 1344).

33. Letter dated 12 January 1867 (Archives of the Provincial House of Rennes, p. 291).

34. Many refused to keep records of toxic substances as categorically ordered by the ordinance of 29 October 1846.

35. Dr. Bijon of Quimperlé, report to the medical society of the department of Finistère, dated 7 May 1861.

36. Council on hygiene of Ploërmel, dated 16 May 1879.

37. Bijon, report. Though no vast sums were involved, certain dispensaries could by this means make as much as a thousand francs a year.

38. Report by the medical board of the department of Loire-Inférieure for the year 1840 (A.D., Loire-Inférieure, 4 X 231).

39. Dr. Gabriel Leborgne, *Le Médecin* (1846), 2: 138-39.

40. Circulating letter by the superior of the sisters of Evron dated 29 May 1858 (A.D., Mayenne, M 1450). The notion of emergencies conveniently cropped up again in a decree dated 14 August 1863 by the high court of appeals, which authorized nuns to bleed and apply leeches in emergencies.

41. Circulating letter of Tirard, minister of agriculture and trade, dated 26 August 1880.

42. Confidential letter by Léon Bourgeois, undersecretary of the interior, dated 1 February 1889.

43. The first associations date from 1881.

44. Dr. L.J.M. Robert, *Manuel de santé* (1805).

45. Prospectus issued by the *Gazette de santé* in 1819.

46. Nuns could even pass on to their propharmacist physician-vassals the wholesale rates given them by druggists and crooked suppliers. Examples are found in the departments of Morbihan, in 1861 (A.D., Morbihan, M 3911), and Mayenne, in 1890 (A.D., Mayenne, M 1452).

47. Letter from the mayor of Ile-aux-Moines, dated 4 May 1859 (A.D., Morbihan, M 991).

48. Becoming a physician in a religious secondary school was an enviable stepping stone in the profession.

49. Doctoral dissertation in medicine, Paris, 1903.

50. Martin, *Précis de déontologie,* p. 55. According to this text, the "intelligent" nuns considered the possibility of a miraculous cure as a rear guard to standard therapy; the nun is shown as siding with the scientist interpretation as far as the "nervous" patient was concerned while abandoning the incurable to their fate.

51. Letter from the prefect of the department of Ille-et-Vilaine, dated 15 October 1818 (A.D., Ille-et-Vilaine, 20 Mk 1).

52. Circulating letter from the bishop of Nantes dated 25 July 1825 (A.D., Loire-Atlantique, 1 M 1344).

53. J.-F. Dervaux, *Le Doigt de Dieu, les filles de la sagesse* (1955), 2: 162.

54. The alliance among medicine, teaching, and religion in the colonies has been studied by Yvonne Turin, *Affrontements culturels dans l'Algérie coloniale (1830-1880)* (Paris: Maspero, 1971).

3

City and Country
in Eighteenth-Century
Medical Discussions
about Early Childhood

Marie-France Morel

The number of medical texts dealing with the "preservation" and "physical education" of children increased considerably during the eighteenth century, especially after the publication of Jean-Jacques Rousseau's *Emile* in 1762. The entire enlightened elite involved in the various academies, learned societies, and salons was interested in this question, which had medical, moral, political, and demographic implications. It was a matter of keeping the maximum number of infants alive during a period when people believed that the population constituted the principal wealth of the state. Physicians were not alone in this fight to save newborn babies. Moralists and theologians, the traditional protectors of childhood, were also interested in early education, as were government administrators, political figures, and philanthropists, all of whom were concerned about increasing the population. Despite this astonishing multiplicity of authors, we are confronted with a debate that is often very full of clichés, with authors copying and plagiarizing one another, and with the same themes being repeated from one work to another. These works argue in favor of the mother's nursing her own child, condemn paid wetnurses, criticize swaddling clothes, and see animal milk as a possible substitute for mother's milk.

In this debate, the contrast between city and country was always an essential point in the argument. Indeed, city children were not raised like those in the country. A quantity of practices set the two groups apart, whether it was a question of nursing, swaddling bands, clothing, weaning, or learning how to

Annales, E. S. C. 32 (September-Oct. 1977): 1007-24. Translated by Patricia M. Ranum.

walk. The physicians, who were writing either for their colleagues or for well-to-do urban families, saw the country as playing an ambiguous role: they viewed it at times as the model to be imitated and at others as the symbol of everything censured by the medical profession. Thus, the city/country dichotomy was applied in both directions, often at only a few pages' interval in the same book. According to the points he was trying to make, the author could cite the healthful and natural education given to country children, or, on the contrary, stigmatize the "routine" and "prejudice" in which such an education was steeped.

Let me stress first that in these debates the city and the country were abstract and idealized places and were always defined in a very vague manner, as if self-evident. Their confines surely were not geographic boundaries. These indefinite spaces were not delineated by city walls. Sociological considerations seem to have been more relevant in a definition. In general, the city was viewed as the residence of rich and cultivated people, whose wealth and social position imposed a special way of life. Parents passed their days and evenings in salons, at balls, or at the theater. Frequently absent, they did little of the actual rearing of their children, who were brought up by a wetnurse at home or sent out to wet-nurse in the country. When the infant remained with its parents, a *remueuse* [a "fidgeter"] came in and attended to all of its physical needs and a *garde* [a "guard"] supervised it during outings. The servants played a very important role in these milieus, and it was often necessary to curtail their bad influence over small children, who were dressed too warmly, clad in clothes that were too tight, and frequently stuffed with goodies. Families of this sort were often mentioned in these volumes by physicians, because they were the very families for whom the books were intended. For the city was the only place where the physician could hope to be read and, on occasion, heeded.

The craftsmen and the lower classes of the city were mentioned occasionally, but with few details (other than their specific ailments); they were generally described as hybrid creatures, country folk and city dwellers at one and the same time. The countryside was seen as essentially inhabited by the poor and the peasants, who lived an exhausting and active life in the open air and raised their children according to practices passed down from generation to generation, not according to medical treatises, which they had never read.

In actual fact, the characteristics that went into the definitions of the city and the country could vary greatly, depending upon the author's argument and the image he was trying to oppose. The city could be either the only place where children were raised in an enlightened manner or a tomb for the unfortunate newborns living there. In like manner, the country could be a totally healthy place for children or, on the contrary, an abyss of barbarism and obscurantism.

These ambivalent contrasts were not limited to medical debates over early childhood. Similar antithetical dichotomies can be found throughout the ideology of the Enlightenment. In anthropology, the savage couple versus the civilized one functioned in an identical way. Sometimes the savage was deprecated in comparison with the civilized man; at others the wretchedness of the social man was contrasted with the happiness of the natural man. "It follows that a single change in image suffices to invert the entire meaning of the discussion."[1] Anthropological explanations were, moreover, always present in the works of authors of treatises dealing with early education. They were very familiar with travel accounts and noted with interest exotic practices concerning suckling or clothing infants. A comparison with savage peoples often provided an argument to incite readers to respect Nature, a major concern of every enlightened education.

Linguistic and ethnological discussions about dialects also show the different and often contradictory use of certain opposites whose meaning could change at the observer's whim: "Passion can be free or savage, speech can be true or vain, simplicity can be worthy of the golden age or quite barbarous, and artifice can be wise or deceitful."[2]

Last, since the Renaissance the definition of the city as the heart of civilization had been reinforced by certain contrasts that showed it to be more worthwhile than the country. "A series of interlocking notations, linked together by means of opposites, spreads this intuition in every direction. It appears in geography, with the antithesis between city and country; in economics, with stability versus progress; in anthropology, with nature versus culture; and in daily life, with rusticity contrasted with urbanity."[3] This definition gradually weakened as the eighteenth century progressed. Picking up the theme first used by the agrarians and then by the physiocrats, moralists and novelists henceforth contrasted the sterility and uselessness of cities with the productivity and virtue of the countryside. In like manner, a body of questions that took shape during the last half of the century led to a study of the various functions of the city and the interdependence of these roles: "Eighteenth-century observers thought they could see, at the heart of the city, a relationship between commerce, industry, and population; mentality and degree of wealth; illnesses and professional activities; and housing and family size."[4] At the end of the century, as a result of the discovery of urban pauperism, this "functional" relationship became linked to the myth about returning to nature. It was the period of the first "emigration" of leading citizens toward the countryside, which was related more to a "new awareness of urban reality" than to "the effect of rustic charms."[5] Discussion about the city therefore remained relatively ambivalent during the eighteenth century. According to their tastes or aspirations, authors laid greater or lesser stress upon the charms and necessary functions of the city by contrasting it with a more or less natural countryside.

Medical debate followed the same pattern, except that it greatly simplified the definitions about the city and presented merely a stereotyped picture. In actual fact, the change in the image of the city/country dichotomy was less important here than the antinomy itself. Above all it was a question of showing that, as far as early upbringing was concerned, city and country were totally different. From the moment when the two were shown to have nothing in common, medical debate could alternately place value upon one or the other.

The Prestige of the City

An initial series of discussions gave preference to the city over the country. This conception developed particularly from sixteenth- and seventeenth-century descriptions of cities. The city was seen as a center of civilization, refinement, and urbanity. This ideal picture of the city reflected both the concrete beauty of its monuments and the culture and morals of its inhabitants. Eighteenth-century physicians continued to use this definition: the city, the center of enlightenment, was contrasted with the cultural desert that was the countryside. Only city dwellers could have the "healthy judgment" and the "enlightened vigilance" needed to preserve the lives of children.[6] Since reason governed all their actions, they were the only ones who listened to physicians' advice. Indeed, in the eighteenth century the city became the only social space with complete medical services, and physicians were writing specifically for those enlightened fathers and mothers whom they often recognized as possessed of a sort of innate knowledge that was in a sense a product of their urban culture. The city was the place where the utopia of a total medicalization of society seemed liable to become a reality. By contrast, in the country, "customs," "prejudice," and ignorance (of good medicine) reigned supreme. It was the perfect example of the seat of nonreason, the domain of pure animality: "The inhabitants of the countryside, whose ideas are as few in number as the objects they desire, have but glimmerings of genius and intelligence; their lives are in most cases as automatic as those of the animals. Once they have finished tilling the soil, they spend the rest of their time drinking and eating."[7]

Hence it was inconceivable that rural women would read medical books in order to learn how to raise their children. They lived in a world where "routine" and old wives' tales were all that counted. Here the city, which already was acculturated by literacy, was contrasted with the country, a region of oral transmission of information, of "belief," and of the irrational:

When a child vomits, without retching, the milk he has just drunk, it is, according to wetnurses, proof that he is in good health, that he is flourishing. They have "heard it said"; and without knowing of what this *so-called* good health consists, they make the fathers and mothers *believe* it. Far from frightening them about the child's health, this dejecta, which is *counter to nature,* reassures them and convinces them that they should once again put the child to the breast.[8]

In reality, for physicians this contrast between urban culture and peasant beliefs was reduced to the fundamental dichotomy of good mother/bad wetnurse. The enlightened mother took physicians' advice; she nursed her own child, refused to put it to wet-nurse, and closely supervised its upbringing. In contrast, women in the country took in strangers' infants in order to earn money. Their feelings were, in the proper sense of the word, *denatured,* since they refused the breast to their own child in order to sell it to a nursling from the city whom they would never love:

Wetnurses can never feel for the child they suckle the powerful instinct that nature has inspired in a mother. Some of them overwhelm the children with caresses in the presence of their mothers; but they are no sooner out of the parents' sight than they treat them like serpents and carry cruelty to the point of beating them, pinching them, throwing them down suddenly, and overwhelming them with curses.[9]

Now, precisely during that period physicians were stressing the importance of an atmosphere of tenderness surrounding the newborn child: "Only a mother's tenderness is capable of that continual vigilance, those necessary little attentions. Can one hope for such tenderness from mercenary and crude wet-nurses?"[10]

The total contrast between the two types of women extended to the smallest detail of early upbringing. The mother's milk was always very suitable for the child, both in quantity and in quality. Nature, "which does everything for the best,"[11] always made sure that the mother's milk would meet her child's needs. The physical qualities of this milk stemmed primarily from the fact that the mother followed the diet prescribed by the physician: "She should eat tender, moist food, nourish herself with soups and meats, eating this at least once a day with a good quantity of soup greens and bread. She should drink only a little wine. . . . She should avoid all bitter, salty, astringent, and above all acid foods, such as leeks, radishes, garlic, salt pork, fatback, cheeses . . . raw fruit, wine, and especially spirits."[12] Thanks to these precautions, the mother's milk would be at the same time good, light, and "serous."

By contrast, rural wetnurses ate a completely different diet. They were fond of the very same "coarse" food of which physicians disapproved, and they ate everything voraciously. Their milk was heavy, difficult to digest, and frequently "heated" by heavy work in the fields. Parents and physicians tried in vain to change these women's eating habits: "We cannot finish this article without confessing some chagrin that, despite the importance of the precepts we have set forth in it concerning the foods that wetnurses should eat, we do not dare to hope that they will be followed, even by a small number. The least change in their routine or their way of life seems impossible for them, or at least pointless."[13] But the physical qualities of the milk were also related to the moral qualities that were transmitted to nurslings with their milk. Good, enlightened mothers gave their children the seeds of the most noble and gentle passions, while wetnurses imparted the worst vices. The physical and moral degeneracy of noble and rich children was caused solely by their having been put out to wet-nurse in the countryside: "So let us conclude that if the children of nobles are degenerate, if the children of the most ingenious individuals become brutish, if the children of the healthiest become feeble and delicate, and if some of them die just as they are beginning to live, the wetnurses most frequently cause all these misfortunes."[14]

After milk came the other foods. Peasant women were capable of weaning their children at an early age and feeding them thick and indigestible porridges as early as their first month of life. "They have been seen to give to their children born a month earlier almost all the foods that they themselves eat."[15] Medical discussions were unanimous on this point. *Coarseness* of food and manners was contrasted with the *lightness* of a diet made up exclusively of milk until the child's second year. *Reason* and the respect for the delicate *nature* of the nursling required weaning it late and slowly, through a "mild, tender, and light" diet based on bread, soups, and clear broths. Moreover, certain authors saw the extreme poverty of the wetnurses as an explanation for the refusal of country people to adopt an intelligent diet: "Most often having no bread for their husbands and their own children, how could one imagine that they would supply food suited to the delicate organs of a nursling; upon weaning, they give them only dry, smoky bread, truffles, chestnuts, and other indigestible foods, which plug the children up and cause them a host of illnesses, such as dehydration, marasmus, dropsy, etc."[16]

Another point against wetnurses was their refusal to give up the use of swaddling clothes. Throughout the seventeenth century, physicians had continued to favor this old custom, because it would assure the child of straight limbs and thus permit him to show himself as distinct from young animals. After 1740, physicians and naturalists on the contrary began to stress the need to respect *Nature,* which would assure a harmonious development for the newborn without recourse to the *artifice* of swaddling bands. The natural beauty of the human body was thus contrasted with the artificial beauty inflicted by style or by routine. What is the natural position assumed by a newborn infant? He tucks his knees up to his chest and his heels against his rump, as he did in the womb: "Thus one is going directly against the desires of that selfsame Nature when one keeps children stretched out and compressed all over in that manner. . . . It is imagined that Nature has refused them the necessary strength to support themselves and that they need the help of art in order to do so."[17]

Here the opposition between nature and art is partly superimposed upon the city/country dichotomy. The swaddling band, an artifice that went contrary "to the laws and intentions of nature,"[18] was a practice created by "the imagination of narrow-minded and coarse people such as paid wetnurses, who had not the slightest knowledge of the natural history of children."[19] In contrast, in certain large cities, swaddling was being done less frequently: "The voice of reason has at last been heard in France. . . . It is above all to the immortal author [Rousseau] of *Emile* that we owe the abolition of the extravagant and barbaric practice of swaddling."[20] This practice continued in rural areas throughout the entire nineteenth century. By 1760 reformers were stressing the difficulty of making wetnurses understand the harm caused by swaddling clothes:

One should expect great opposition from wetnurses, to whom a tightly wrapped child gives less trouble than one who must be continually watched. Besides, a loose garment makes it more noticeable that the child has soiled itself; he must be cleaned up more often. In short, in certain regions the custom is an argument that will never be refuted to the satisfaction of people of all estates.[21]

Using various names (custom, prejudice, ignorance, routine), medical discussions during the Enlightenment stigmatized the resistance shown by peasant wetnurses to the rational innovations proposed by urban physicians. The latter realized vaguely that their precepts clashed with a very powerful body of popular knowledge that provided all the coherence underlying the procedures followed by country women. They persistently refused to accept this coherence as a fact and condemned wetnurses wholesale in the name of the superiority of their erudite culture.

Along with swaddling, the cleanliness of the infant was one of the chief battlefields of this confrontation between two opposing bodies of knowledge. In the eighteenth century, scholarly medicine stressed how important personal hygiene was to the maintenance of health. Illness, in some of its manifestations, was caused by the perspiration and filth that seeped back into the body as a poison. Hence the importance of daily baths for children, which physicians recommended strongly from this time on: "The foundation of health is the regularity with which perspiration occurs. . . . In order to attain this important point, children must be washed a few days after their birth in cold water, such as that fetched from the spring. . . . They must be washed very regularly every day, no matter what the weather or the season of the year."[22] The benefits of the bath were moral as much as physical, hence the use of cold water. It was less a matter of washing the child than of toughening him from his earliest days by giving him a well-"tempered" character [as iron is tempered by dipping it in cold water].

This harsh upbringing, which in some respects was almost rustic, was not at all appreciated by the peasants. All physicians stressed how difficult it was to convince them. And so, although one of these physicians bathed his son every day in cold water throughout several cold winters, his example aroused little but curiosity and criticism from the peasants of Picardy among whom he lived: "My son became the object of the curiosity and wonder of the entire region where, far from adopting my principles of physical education, on the basis of an example of this sort, they said I was very lucky that my son had stood up to everything I had done to kill him."[23]

Popular behavior, on the contrary, stressed the necessary precautions to be taken when disposing of excrement or removing body dirt. One should not wash too often or wash all parts of the body indiscriminately, for dirt was a part of the body and in a certain way played a protective role, especially for the child, who was more exposed to evil spirits than the adult. Hence, the relative filth in which many nurslings were kept, a filth that was severely criticized by physicians: "One must wash behind their ears and their entire head, taking care not to press upon the fontanelle, and brush the head often, in order to prevent the formation of what wetnurses call the "cradle cap." This filth is not at all necessary, no matter what they say."[24] Here again, the physicians were attributing these procedures to the laziness or ignorance of wetnurses, without understanding the strength in rural areas of the symbolic system that placed a value upon filth.[25] The gap between urban and rural practices widened, because hygiene was beginning to become a major concern for urban governments and public baths and private bathrooms were beginning to make their appearance in cities.

The physicians' insistence can be explained by the importance of the stakes: the survival of urban infants, almost all of whom were entrusted to "mercenary" wetnurses. All authors stressed the "depopulation" for which these women were responsible. "Infinitely more children die through the abuses of wetnurses than for any other cause."[26] But could wetnurses really be "enlightened"? The majority of physicians were so convinced of these women's ignorance and stupidity that they despaired ever changing their habits. In vain, parents tried to impose upon them the rules prescribed by physicians; the nurses would promise to do everything asked but would resume "their old ways" as soon as they had returned to their village. On several occasions parents were able to catch them in their irrational and routine practices. The only solution was to take the wetnurse away from her rural home in order to keep her "always under your eyes . . . at home,"[27] in the city. But such a solution was feasible only for those households that were wealthy enough and adequately enough housed to permit keeping a wetnurse at home.

Foundlings were especially vulnerable, above all when put to wet-nurse in the countryside. At the end of the Ancien Régime, every hospital administrator stressed the frighteningly high death rate, which was attributed on the one hand to the natural weakness of these children, owing to the very conditions surrounding their birth and abandonment, and on the other to bad wetnurses. Indeed, the hospitals of the day, which found themselves burdened with an increasing number of infants, could only place them in the poorest villages, in the homes of the most poverty-stricken wetnurses. This dramatic situation gradually gave rise to the idea that the lives of more children would be saved if they were kept in the city under medical surveillance. Thus, in 1789 the town council of Caen firmly proposed a solution confirming the superiority of the city in matters of early education. "The bastards of Caen, suckled on the spot, are much better cared for, more healthy, and more robust than those in the countryside."[28] This new awareness lay behind numerous experiments in artificial feeding attempted in foundling hospitals during the late eighteenth century under the supervision of physicians and surgeons.[29]

Nonetheless, a few physicians did not give up hope of educating rural women. Gilibert, of Lyons, paid regular visits to some thirty wetnurses during the 1760s and noted that the infant mortality rate was decreasing. In Picardy, Fourcroy de Guillerville taught peasant men how to dress children as lightly as possible, even during the coldest days of winter. Note that initially only the men were invited to attend this lesson in child care. They naively showed amazement at the physician's knowledge; and when the doctor later told the story, he gave himself the starring role. The use of a few popular expressions in his text lends emphasis to the infinite distance separating medical knowledge from popular practices:

They remained enraptured and said to one another: "We would never dare tell those women what we sees here, they would say that we's lied, but is true. They takes so much trouble to keep th' children warm, to swaddle 'em, to keep 'em bundled up; and still their feet's always like ice. But here, where they's no fire, and they's almost naked, is warm as toast. How can that be?" By dint of giving them reasons within their comprehension, and above all by endoctrinating the women who come to consult me, I managed to get a lot of them to stop swaddling their infants, whom they keep less warm and no longer are so concerned with protecting from the cold. That is all for the better for those little wretches.

And thus, by imperceptible degrees, good practices can spread and become established for the good of humanity. Once the opinions of the common people have been changed by repeated examples that always reinforce the method I am proposing, my method can become universal. But above all they need examples, and it is up to level-headed and unprejudiced individuals to provide those examples.[30]

Indeed, physicians could see only one reasonable way of raising children, the one they were proposing, which was based upon a multitude of very strict and obligatory principles: "You should feed [your child], warm it, clean it of the dirt it brings with it at birth and the dirt to which it is subject daily. You must dress it, see that it sleeps deeply, ease its pains. All these goals demand a host of essential precautions. Omit one of them and you are threatened with the loss of your child. Together they take a mother out of herself and make her the slave of her nursling."[31] It was useless to hope that country women, "ignorant" and overwhelmed with heavy work, would pay such close attention to all these little details. Because early child rearing had become an increasingly medical subject at the end of the eighteenth century, it became a characteristically urban concern. With the final success of scholarly medicine, "a secondary effect of urban supremacy,"[32] country ways were censured.

The Charm of the Country

During the years when the preeminence of the city in matters of early childhood was developing, an increasingly larger number of authors were showing that children could no longer be raised there safely. Physicians contributed medical arguments to the literary and economic movement praising the virtues of the countryside in contrast to the corruption of the cities. Here again the contrast was as much physical as moral.

All physicians stressed first of all the poor quality of city air. Even in well-aired neighborhoods, the air was always impure and bore within it the chief cause of all urban illnesses. Country air was, on the other hand, the subject of glowing descriptions:

The morning air brings to the person who inhales it a strength and a well-being the effects of which he feels all day long. The exhalations from the soil, at the moment when the plow opens new furrows; from the dew, which is the sap of the plants, a sort of volatile balm; from the flowers, never as perceptible as at daybreak, are all causes that give those who enjoy country air, under these various circumstances, a life principle that is absolutely lacking for those who never inhale anything but the air in rooms. . . . The moving air to which the peasant is often exposed is another one of the major causes of his strength and health.[33]

The importance of air as a cause of all illnesses—a commonplace in the medical thought of the day—can be found in every treatise on early childhood. To a greater degree than the adult, the child was sensitive to the good and bad effects of the air. Several physicians even stressed that country air all by itself was sufficient to cure small children of childhood ailments, such as teething, which generally coincided with weaning and the early return of urban children to their parents:

The pure and bracing air inhaled in the fields is singularly influential in promoting this important and critical function of nature; . . . it is an error to cause children, during this period, to pass from this elastic and healthful air to the air of the city, and above all a large city, where the air has lost its most healthful and most praiseworthy qualities; this reason should be a consideration in not removing children from the countryside so soon.[34]

Even the physicians most in favor of maternal nursing admitted that putting to wet-nurse at least had the advantage of removing the child from the miasmas of the big city. "This stay [in the country] is the only thing that compensates somewhat for their not having been nursed by their mothers."[35] The majority of authors, therefore, drew the logical conclusion that "of any given number, more children die in the city than in the country."[36] Only a few, like Ballexserd, were sufficiently hostile to putting an infant to wet-nurse to assert that "by itself good air is not sufficient to maintain health and preserve children."[37]

Thus, physicians can be seen as the popularizers of the physiocrats' ideas concerning the superiority of the country over the city. In their discussions the cities are shown as centers of luxury, corruption, and declining population; the countryside as the source of all wealth, both agricultural and demographic, for there the women are more fertile and the children more robust. Thanks to the peasants, the state would be more populous, more wealthy, and better served. Medical precepts about early child rearing only assume their full meaning when they are seen in relationship to this ideology, which had spread to so much of the elite of the Enlightenment. Indeed, the economic and demographic contrast was basically a moral one. In the city people led sedentary, inactive lives that went against nature; they spent their time eating, gambling, dancing, and partying far into the night. In contrast, the peasants led an active, simple, and virtuous life, which brought them joy and health. The country man, "awoke and put to bed with the sun, enjoys all the advantages that the presence of that star on the horizon gives to the atmosphere."[38] He lived in a natural manner. Even better, he *was nature,* and he showed it in every facet of his way of life. It was because he respected nature that he was endowed with robust health. According to Tissot, there was a relationship between the various ways of life and the degree of health. Healthiness gradually and regularly decreased as one approached the city. The healthiest people of all were the savages,

who know nothing of most ailments and who only die from accidents or decrepitude. To the degree that one moves away from their estate, health seems to decline by degrees. Our *laboureurs* [independent farmers] are less healthy than they, because they do not live exclusively the life of the fields: some of them have been domestic servants, others soldiers. They have weakened their health in these two occupations and have brought to their villages some of the customs of the city.

The closer one approached the city, the clearer the relationship between geography and typology of health. The middle classes "already show many ailments unknown in the country." Those most to be pitied were the "society folk," who were distinguished by the idleness and excesses of that life style. They were often stricken by "ailments that are almost unknown to villagers,"[39] owing to an overly rich diet, staying up until the wee hours, lack of exercise, tight-fitting clothes, excessive recourse to the pleasures of love at an early age, and overly ardent passions. In contrast, the peasant, typified by a great "economy of ideas," always enjoyed good health, "which almost always is in inverse proportion to the faculties of the mind."[40] This natural vigor was especially evident in peasant women: "What a difference between the strength and health of village girls and of young ladies! Why do the former have such good color, rosy cheeks, and a constitution unaffected by all the vicissitudes of the seasons, while the latter drag out wretched lives, always languid and prostrated by the least bit of intemperate weather?"[41]

Medicine of the period was in the process of discovering new illnesses to which women were prone: fainting, vapors, languishing—"female protective behavior" resulting from the moral crisis in marital values among well-to-do urban families.[42] These ailments had major consequences for the health of newborn infants. Urban women frequently experienced difficult pregnancies and then had trouble nursing their children, even when they wished to do so. "If they nurse, without the care required by this new estate, they become exhausted and fall into a nervous ailment."[43] Their antinatural way of life, and above all the excessive passions they experienced daily, altered their milk. In the best of cases, they could only offer their children a "heated" milk that was not very nourishing and that led to the infant's death. If they gave up the idea of nursing, their own life was endangered, for their milk was reabsorbed into the body and, in flowing, "gives rise to an infinity of ailments, almost all of them unfortunate and difficult to cure. Among them, there is a very sad one, since it works to the detriment of the population. To date no one has discussed this ailment. It is a sort of paralysis of the uterus, as a result of the loss of milk, which makes these women insensitive to pleasure and unable to conceive."[44]

Country women, on the contrary, were robust by nature. "Paid wetnurses

. . . are part of an order of which good health is almost always a part."[45] Like the cows they raised, they always gave excellent milk; and this milk transmitted a bit of their robustness to the weak city child. Having only simple and rustic passions, they were less likely to transmit them to the children they nursed. A hierarchy of milks corresponded to the hierarchy of passions. Simple and rustic passions did not alter the good milk of country women, but the violent passions of society women poisoned their ethereal milk. Hence the idea of correcting the innate weakness of city children by means of animal milk, which was even closer to nature, more regular, and free from passions: "The milk of animals is not subject to the same drawbacks as that of women. Their way of life is uniform, their food always the same, or similar, and their instinct keeps them from anything that might harm them."[46] The experiments with artificial feeding of newborns conducted during the eighteenth century were carried out for two motives. They either stemmed from a theoretical idea —carried to the extreme—that the countryside and beneficent nature (of which animals were a part) were the source of all health or else they were prompted by the need to save the lives of more children, by no longer putting them to wet-nurse and by having them supervised in the city by physicians.

Given the theoretical possibility of using animal milk, certain writers began to daydream. Baldini, an Italian, hoped to find the means of correcting the distinctive natures of city and country children. Children from the city, he said, have "a melancholy temperament; they are dull, lazy, and their minds are overwhelmed by the weight of their humors." Goat's milk would give their minds "more life" and "more penetration." On the other hand, cow's milk would be more suitable for peasant children, "born of a father and mother who lead active lives, who are strong and lively. By this means one could modify the rapid flow of their humors; they would be made less ingenious, more substantial."[47] In like vein, other authors proposed correcting the various national characteristics by choosing an animal whose milk was the opposite of each nation's weaknesses: goat's milk for the Germans, cow's milk for the Italians.

The quality of the milk was not the only factor that distinguished the nurslings raised in the city from those raised in the country. The urban way of life was also held responsible for the numerous physical deformities found in the children of well-to-do families. Indeed, although swaddling was an almost universal practice (until criticism by the medical profession resulted in a slight decline at the end of the eighteenth century), only people who were "above the ordinary" forced their small children—as early as their first birthday—to wear a sort of corset made with very stiff whalebone stays to ensure that, while learning to walk, they would stand straight, a posture deemed more appropriate to their estate (crawling being curbed as "animallike"). They were also eager to make sure that young children (both boys and girls) would have elegant and graceful bodies that fit the norms dictated by the styles of the day. Thin waists and flat bellies were physical signs that a child came of a good family: "They seek solely to give them an elegant torso; they are concerned with shaping their bodies so that their shoulders slope, their arms are pulled back, their spines are prefectly straight, their necks long, their waists thin, their hips low, and their bellies flat."[48]

According to parents, these very constraining aesthetic norms would never be attained if children were allowed to grow up freely. If care was not taken during their childhood years to begin to mold their bodies by means of all the resources available through "art," "children will relax and, no longer receiving support, will become humpbacked and misshapen; they will have high shoulders, they will be neckless; girls will have monstrous bellies and will no longer dare to appear in public."[49] Physicians condemned this disastrous practice and held it responsible for the countless deformities they had noted in city women: "Narrow hips, heavy shoulders, twisted spines, and flat, thin, and compressed chests are the special attributes of the city dweller, especially among the bourgeoisie and the well-to-do."[50]

This unsatisfactory physical conformation, provoked by the wearing of whalebone corsets, was also responsible for very frequent miscarriages and for malformed breasts, which often made nursing impossible: "The compression experienced by the breasts during childhood not only weakens them but destroys their tips; an infinite number of newborn children die because their mothers' breasts have no nipples. At the very best, they are in such poor condition, so small and weak, that most mothers who nurse suffer considerably from inflammations and breast abscesses."[51] But stylish concerns did not exist for country girls or for those from the urban lower classes:

Their financial situation or the need to work do not permit them to wear corsets. How many of them are, we note, very erect, with shapely bodies, and even pretty! On the contrary, how many of those who remove their corsets only at bedtime are seen to be missshapen, humpbacked, or thick waisted, with uneven hips, one jutting out more than the other! The corset is not absolutely necessary for giving girls the inestimable merit of possessing a shapely body. Let them put a bit more trust in the operations of nature, let them strive to foster the uniformity and consistency of those operations, and we have no doubts about assuring them great success.[52]

The arguments made by physicians consisted of showing parents that Nature always did things well and that she had created people to stand erect. Thus, no tampering with the child's physical development should obstruct her from completing her work in the child. Only peasants and savages were capable of this; city people lived against nature. This was why the physiological obstacles to nursing seemed to occur far more frequently among well-born women than among country ones. The peasant woman rarely was humpbacked, she always had a generous bosom, and her body was naturally better adapted to pregnancy and lactation.[53] Thus, we see two contrasting types of human body: the one found in the city and the one found in the country. The superiority of the rural body was confirmed by everything involving physical and moral health.

The conclusion to be drawn from this repeated contrast between urban and rural child rearing appeared clear to physicians. If the mothers were indeed different in their physical appearance, their children were no less so. "What an enormous difference can be observed between country children, who know how to run and jump by the age of two, and our city children, who can scarcely walk at two or three years of age!"[54]

Inactivity, indolence, and bad health were the lot of the wretched city child; activity, liveliness, robustness, and health were reserved for the children of peasants. These differences became accentuated after weaning. The parents in well-to-do families kept their children fragile by underfeeding them. They did not want their offspring to become fat and healthy, "because they say that resembles the peasant too closely."[55] Through their concern with showing that their children were a race apart from country children, certain parents almost let them die of hunger. In the country, on the contrary, people liked fat children and prized plumpness for its esthetic value. Thus, they tended to overfeed children (when possible) in order to show that they were "thriving." While they criticized the practice of stuffing children with coarse gruels, physicians realized that peasant children were often better nourished and digested food more easily than their urban counterparts.

Though the country was the ideal place for good health, all city dwellers should not, however, be encouraged to live like peasants. Physicians were careful to show that it was impossible to eliminate the differences between two totally different milieus. They were eager to maintain the ailments to which city folk were prone as specifically urban ones and used cultural and social factors as arguments:

I do not invite you to live like the savages, who, in the main prey to stupid indolence from which they almost never arouse themselves other than to hunt or seek revenge, lead the life of the carnivorous animal rather than that of the rational being. Nor do I urge you back to the life of the plowman, although I believe that in actual fact his life is happier than that of the man of the world. But two classes of very marked pleasures, which are derived from the cultivation of the mind and the exercise of the feelings, are almost lost to the plowman and contribute powerfully to increase the happiness of the man who enjoys them.[56]

Desessartz gave more concrete advice, suggesting that city women exercise and refrain from placing their children in whalebone corsets. In order to be heeded, he felt it necessary to reassure his auditors about his true intentions: "Distinctions in rank and social station are a wise and necessary institution for the happiness of society, and, in recommending that women exercise, we are far from intending to disparage them to the point of obliging them to share field work with peasant women."[57]

Thus, medical discussions about early child rearing were discussions about differences. They were inspired by the same ideology as the other debates of the period and, like them, stressed the irreducible inequality between city and country. As one physician stated in his reply to Grégoire's inquiry about local dialects, it was a matter of "two peoples," who were totally different.[58] The peasant was the Other Person, the Savage, who was at one and the same time the model and the foil, the near relative and the distant kin of the city dweller.

Indeed, according to whether they were given a negative or a positive connotation, the terms city and country referred to different realities. When the city was extolled at the expense of the countryside, the contrast was based upon the difference between the enlightened, good mother and the paid, routine-minded wetnurse. Or, when the countryside was praised, it was a question of stressing the dichotomies bad health/good health and artifice/ nature by opposing the society world and the peasantry. The debates of the Enlightenment, therefore, functioned through contrasting, term by term, two series of lists. One was a list of behavior (nurse one's child, sell one's milk) and the other was a list of social conditions (the artificial life of the city, the natural life of the peasantry). The former was based upon *doing,* the latter upon *being.* These ways of behaving or ways of life were attributed to the social roles that, in these discussions, were sometimes shown as personages (the good mother or the bad wetnurse), and at others as ways of life (urban versus city life). As a result, these antagonistic roles served as supports for two systems of contrasting values. It was sufficient simply to invert the values, and the enlightened mother, who had been contrasted with the prejudiced wet-nurse, became the worldly city dweller who served as a foil for the natural country woman. The regular use of these series of paradigms made it possible for the medical debate to proceed as it did.

In reality, there was a profound inequality between physicians' knowledge of the city and their knowledge of the country. Even more than an inequality in information or experience, their summary presentation of the countryside doubtlessly involved a simplification of their vague ideas about the knowledge of the common people in order to serve the aspects of urban medical knowledge they wanted to show as superior. And so the contrast that seems to give equal roles to the city and the country was no more equitable when it placed value upon the country than when it discredited it. In this instance, parallelism and antithesis were the instruments of power.

Certain more clear-sighted physicians, such as members of the Société Royale de Médecine, occasionally refused to use this rhetoric. For them neither the city nor the country was an ideal place to raise children. The city had become an unhealthy place, and the natural countryside no longer existed because urban manners had spread to the rural areas and had corrupted them. Thus, the city itself was responsible for the abuses of which the rural wetnurses were so vehemently accused: "Since city women seek wetnurses among country women, the latter abandon their infants to sell their milk to children who are total strangers. This is how the damage spreads, and how a denatured mother casts guilt upon another mother, who, but for her, would have heeded the *voice of her blood and of nature.*"[59]

Above all, these physicians were discovering the extreme poverty of the countryside, which explained why women found it advantageous to sell their milk so cheaply. They were also familiar with the ailments and poor health of most peasants. They attributed poverty to the excessive tax burden and called upon the government to improve the condition of the peasantry. This involved broadening the physicians' sphere of activity to the entire rural area and to all social classes. Physicians did not wish to be heeded solely in the city; they also wanted to put in a word about the health and happiness of country people, especially children:

> The great mass of the inhabitants of Europe can be divided into three orders or classes of citizens. The first is made up of the great and the rich; the second of bourgeois and artisans; and, by custom more than by reason, the third is apportioned among the peasants or the poor inhabitants of the countryside. Now, what is the manner of existence, the sort of life, and the posterity born of the one and the other groups?
>
> The children of the first group, feeble products of men who are degenerate or barely formed, share their parents' vices and expiate the mistakes of the entire species. Those of the second group, raised in confined quarters and nourished among black vapors or poisonous fumes, are already more feeble at birth [than the rich or the great], and those seeds of illness that they bear at their birth grow daily in a poisoned atmosphere. As for the poor inhabitants of the country (who are besieged on all sides by exhorbitant taxes, who encounter endless red tape when paying them, and who by paying them are deprived of physical necessities and, before that, of spiritual calm), they often water with their tears a soil that their weakened arms can no longer till. These sapless branches bear no new shoots, but merely sterile, languishing ones that die soon after they sprout. The great and the rich should therefore be raised in a simpler and more virile manner and should decide marriages under the patronage of love and innocence rather than that of convenience, which is used to mask foolish pride or greedy self-interest. Our cities should no longer be allowed to overflow with people piled one atop the other and bent over a thousand minor trades, which give them specific ailments belonging only to their craft and to their puny posterity. Last, the heads of nations, the arbiters of political societies, should be willing to sense clearly that wherever the common people are happy, the population is numerous and that on the contrary, everything dries up, everything languishes and flickers out as a result of oppression and constraint.[60]

NOTES

1. Michèle Duchet, *Anthropologie et histoire au siècle des Lumières* (Paris, 1971), p. 11.

2. Michel de Certeau, Dominique Julia, and Jacques Revel, *Une Politique de la lange. La Révolution française et le patois: L'Enquête de Grégoire* (Paris, 1975), p. 153.

3. J.-C. Perrot, *Genèse d'une ville moderne: Caen au XVIIIe siècle* (Paris, 1975), p. 10.

4. Ibid., p. 12.

5. Ibid., p. 26.

6. J. Ballexserd, *Dissertation sur cette question: Quelles sont les cause principales de la mort d'un aussi grand nombre d'enfans . . . ?* (Geneva, 1775), p. 64.

7. J. E. Gilibert, *Dissertation sur la dépopulation causée par les vices, les préjugés et les erreurs des nourrices mercenaires* (Lyons, 1770), p. 299. All discussions during the Enlightenment about the peasants stressed the analogy between the country person and animals: "The peasant who has no possessions of his own (and the majority of them are that way), being as lazy as the oxen which he works and spends his life, scarcely thinks about anything but what he sees and touches" (quoted by de Certeau, Julia, and Revel, *Une Politique de la langue,* p. 149).

8. J. C. Desessartz, *Traité de l'éducation corporelle des enfans en bas-âge, ou réflexions pratiques sur les moyens de procurer une meilleure constitution aux citoyens,* 2nd ed. (Paris,

1799), pp. 211-12. The italics are mine. A few pages later (p. 215), the author criticizes "the chimerical trust wetnurses have that gruel will calm colic."

9. Karl von Linné, *La Nourrice marâtre . . .*, French translation (Lyons, 1770), p. 239.

10. Buffon, *Histoire naturelle* (Paris, 1749), 2: 460.

11. J. Ballexserd, *Dissertation sur l'éducation physique des enfans, depuis leur naissance jusqu'à l'âge de puberté* (Paris, 1767), p. 71.

12. Desessartz, *Traité*, pp. 193-94.

13. Ibid., p. 195.

14. Von Linné, *La Nourrice marâtre*, pp. 243-44.

15. J. Caillau, *Avis aux mères de famille sur l'éducation physique et les maladies des enfans, depuis le moment de leur naissance jusqu'à l'âge de six ans* (Bordeaux, 1797), p. 59.

16. Gilibert, *Dissertation sur la dépopulation*, p. 288.

17. J. L. Fourcroy de Guillerville, *Les Enfants dans l'ordre de la nature ou abrégé de l'histoire naturelle des enfants du premier âge à l'usage des pères et mères de famille* (Paris, 1774), pp. 33, 144.

18. J. P. Frank, *Traité sur la manière d'élever sainement les enfans*, French translation (Paris, 1799), p. 114.

19. Fourcroy de Guillerville, *Les Enfants*, p. 144.

20. Gaillau, *Avis aux mères*, pp. 9-10. This evidence for Bordeaux also applies to Paris. Cf. Sebastien Mercier, *Tableau de Paris* (Amsterdam, 1782-83), 2: 225, "They have adopted the fortunate habit of dressing them lightly and without bands."

21. Jean-Jacques Rousseau, *Emile, ou de l'education*, Pléiade editions (The Hague, 1762), p. 279.

22. S. A. Tissot, *Avis au peuple sur sa santé* (Lausanne, 1771), pp. 390-91.

23. Fourcroy de Guillerville, *Les Enfants*, p. 81.

24. Madame Le Rebours, *Avis aux mères qui veulent nourrir leurs enfans* (Paris, 1767), p. 215.

25. For an explanation of popular knowledge about early child rearing, see F. Loux and Marie-France Morel, "L'Enfance et les savoirs sur le corps: Pratiques médicales et pratiques populaires dans la France traditionnelle," *Ethnologie française* (1976).

26. F. Baldini, *Manière d'allaiter les enfans à la main, au défaut de nourrices*, French translation (Paris, 1788), p. 52.

27. Desessartz, *Traité*, p. 195.

28. Quoted by Perrot, *Genèse d'une ville moderne*, p. 852.

29. On this question see Marie-France Morel, "Théories et pratiques de l'allaitement en France au XVIIIe siècle," *Annales de démographie historique* (1976).

30. Fourcroy de Guillerville, *Les Enfants*, pp. 112-14.

31. Gilibert, *Dissertation sur la dépopulation*, p. 260.

32. Perrot, *Genèse d'une ville moderne*, p. 853.

33. S. A. Tissot, *Essai sur les maladies des gens du monde* (Lausanne, 1770), pp. 25-6. This same emphasis on the therapeutic virtues of morning air can be found in Moheau, *Recherches et considérations sur la population de la France* (Paris, 1778), 2: 111:

> Breathing the morning air, that balm of the senses, that natural medicine, that purest food, is not available to a great part of society; there are a great number of men and women who are not familiar with the dawn or who have only seen it after their sensations have been weakened by the fatigues of nocturnal pleasures. What childhood is to life, what springtime is to the year, the dawn is to the day; and it is a fertile life principle, newly consecrated at the moment of its appearance: the healthy man feels its fortunate effects, and the sick man, exhausted by his suffering, cannot resume living and dies at that time. Must the most refined nation as far as tastes are concerned, the nation that is the most avid for fresh produce, be disdainful and neglectful of one of those products that is the most delicious, perhaps because it is easier to enjoy?

34. Ballexserd, *Dissertation sur cette question*, p. 83.

35. Ibid., p. 83.

36. Tissot, *Avis au peuple*, p. 10. The same conclusions were drawn by Deparcieux, *Essai sur les probabilités de la durée de la vie humaine* (Paris, 1746).

37. Ballexserd, *Dissertation sur cette question*, p. 84.

38. Tissot, *Essai sur les maladies*, p. 24.

39. Ibid., pp. 10-12. Concerning this same text, see also Michel Foucault, *Naissance de la clinique: Une Archéologie du regard médical* (Paris, 1963), p. 16: illness is the most "natural"

in the countryside. "But the more complex the social space in which it is situated becomes, the more *denatured* [illness] becomes."

40. Tissot, *Essai sur les maladies*, p. 32.

41. Desessartz, *Traité*, p. 341.

42. Perrot, *Genèse d'une ville moderne*, p. 834.

43. Tissot, *Essai sur les maladies*, p. 54.

44. Ibid., p. 54.

45. N. Brouzet, *Essai sur l'éducation médicinale des enfants et sur leurs maladies* (Paris, 1754), 1: 171.

46. J. Raulin, *De la conservation des enfants, ou les moyens de les fortifier, de les préserver et guérir des maladies, depuis l'instant de leur existence, jusqu'à l'âge de la puberté* (Paris, 1768-9), 2: 305-6.

47. Baldini, *Manière d'allaiter*, pp. 77-79.

48. Raulin, *De la conservation*, 2: 258.

49. Desessartz, *Traité*, p. 322.

50. Fourcroy de Guillerville, *Les Enfants*, p. 43.

51. B. C. Faust, . . . *sur un vêtement libre, uniforme, national à l'usage des enfans* (1792), p. 14.

52. Desessartz, *Traité*, pp. 322-23.

53. Indeed, Tissot emphasized that city girls menstruated earlier than country ones and during their whole life remained weakened by the precosity and irregularity of their periods. On the contrary, "although their periods begin late among country girls, they are much more regular; the uniformity of their life creates for them the greatest order in this respect, and this order contributes greatly to their good health" (*Essai sur les maladies*, pp. 77-78).

54. Desessartz, *Traité*, p. 341.

55. Ballexserd, *Dissertation sur l'éducation physique*, p. 125.

56. Tissot, *Essai sur les maladies*, pp. 99-100.

57. Desessartz, *Traité*, p. 356.

58. Quoted in de Certeau, Julia, and Revel, *Une Politique de la langue*, p. 153.

59. Charles White, *Avis aux femmes enceintes et en couches ou traité des moyens de prévenir et de guérir les maladies qui les affligent dans ces deux états*, translated from English and expanded in *Traité sur l'allaitement maternel* (Paris, 1774), p. 125. The italics are mine.

60. Ballexserd, *Dissertation sur cette question*, pp. 4-5. See also, for the relationships between ideology and history, Claude Lefort, "L'Ere de l'idéologie," *Encyclopaedia Universalis, Organum*, p. 82: In the ideology of the bourgeoisie "to the degree that the question arises of how the social was engendered from its proper place—the control of that procreation and the ways of refusing to give it recognition and of containing it being lacking—a new type of discussion appears, *concerned with disarming opposition and ruptures within the double register of space and time*. Put in other terms, the ideology is the linking of representations whose function it is to *restore the dimension of the 'historyless' society within the very bosom of the historical society.*"

4

Talent, Reason, and Sacrifice: The Physician during the Enlightenment

Daniel Roche

The Société Royale de Médecine, the last-born of the great Parisian academies, inherited the procedures and customs that had gradually been developed and defined by the older institutions.[1] It seemed perfectly natural for Vicq D'Azyr [perpetual general secretary for the society] to adopt one of these procedures, the academic eulogy. Indeed, for over a century, paying homage to deceased members had been indispensable to the scientific and literary world. Disseminated and read in the provinces and abroad, these eulogies provided an incomparable source of information and a unifying factor, even though they gave rise to a movement critical of the laudatory and rhetorical abuses of the genre. The new Société Royale de Médecine adopted for its own purposes a collective procedure that was appreciated by the entire world of the academies; in doing so it became part of a harmonious framework within which, through its various functions, the genre of the eulogy defined some of the characteristic thought patterns of members of the various academies, that is, of the cultural and political elites. Yet the Société Royale gave to these eulogies a special tone all its own. Within the academic world was a medical subgroup that is extremely interesting to analyze regarding the immediate significance of the innovations sought by the Société Royale and the medical situation of the time as perceived by those physicians who were members of the group or who supported its aims. Insofar as the Société Royale was a harbinger of a profound change in the practice of medicine,[2] it is a matter of interest to study at its source the manner in which the various protagonists in this transformation perceived and described their activities.

Annales, E. S. C. 32 (September-October 1977): 866-86. Translated by Patricia M. Ranum.

The documents make such a study possible. From 1776 to 1789, Vicq d'Azyr delivered about fifty eulogies[3] during public ceremonies of the society, eulogies subsequently published in the *Mémoires de la Société Royale de Médecine*. After 1778 the general secretary reprinted selected eulogies and distributed them to his collaborators in the provinces, among them Hugues Maret.[4] These eulogies show great consistency, for they were edited by a single author and include chiefly physicians[5] or practitioners of a medical profession. In all, forty-five physicians, three physician-surgeons, three surgeons, and three apothecaries and chemists were eulogized. Although these fifty-odd cases cannot be claimed as representative of the entire medical profession, or even of all the regular correspondents of the Société Royale, they provide both enough diversity and enough coherence to permit me to sketch the collective profile of the French medical elite, viewed at its summit. The usual portrait of the physician during the Enlightenment—the genius teaching in the great scholarly institutions of France or Europe or the humble provincial surgeon responsible for providing care during epidemics— appears to some degree here, in the pattern of thought if not the ideology; for the researcher is not confronted with the actual social situation, but rather its multiple refraction and distortion as it is reflected in the mirror of the eulogy. That is why, before turning to the rough portrait of a model physician, with his civic and humanitarian norms, his cultural codes, and his scholarly notes, we must first look at how Vicq d'Azyr initially interpreted the traditional eulogy and then look at the specific functions around which the general secretary of the Société Royale de Médecine, surely more or less consciously, oriented the way in which the genre would habitually be used. The play of light and shadow cast by funeral rhetoric may permit us to uncover both the aspirations of the group of medical innovators and the social and political goals of the government administrators who supported their undertaking. "In order to preserve the memory of the services rendered by the members of the society, it was decided that details concerning their lives and work would be included in our volumes, in the form of either commentaries or eulogies, according to the acknowledged merit of their authors. In order to avoid any excess in this genre, the society will confer this honor after debate in one of its assemblies."[6]

This administrative-sounding text is found at the end of the history of the first years of the Société Royale, immediately after the alphabetical list of the illustrious dead of the year and immediately before the first eulogy published by Vicq d'Azyr. It set a precedent. Like all the scholarly societies, the Académie de Médecine was expected to pay the last honors to its members. The text specifies the manner in which this should be done and defines its limits: it was to be a collective act, emanating from a deliberative assembly that weighed the merits and values of the "services rendered." Exaggeration must be avoided, yet each should receive his due. As spokesman for the academy, the perpetual secretary, who was appointed for life, deplored a death and proclaimed for eternity a judgment of the man and his work, the personage and the person, his work and his morals. The assembly would see itself reflected in this speaker and in the member in whose memory the eulogy was given.

The custom of presenting a eulogy thus combines three functions. The first is rhetorical and is less concerned with the true biographical eulogy than with the manner in which it is expressed; the second is documentary and cognitive, postulating a truth through a description of what is by definition an exemplary history; and the third is hagiographic and imposes a world vision, promotes an ethic, and instills an ideology. These three roles closely overlap in the speeches, even when one or another of them seems to predominate; and this very choice became the focus of the discussions that pitted the partisans of the "oratorical" speech against those who were concerned with the "historical" record, "in order to serve the history of letters, of which truth should be the principal characteristic."[7] On this point Vicq d'Azyr shared the ideas of Thomas and d'Alembert, repeated and amplified by their Parisian followers Dussault, Delisle de Salles, and Lacretelle. So it was a question of denouncing laudatory rhetoric and apologetic amplification and of defending the philosophical lesson intended for *educated* listeners—and readers—who were capable of grasping the progress achieved by the individual being discussed in the history of letters and sciences, and for *philosophic* listeners, that is, individuals capable of understanding the moral value of a life that bore witness to the respectability of intellectuals and that therefore justified their talents and merits. Heir of Fontenelle, Duclos, Buffon, and Voltaire, the general secretary of the Société Royale de Médecine used prosopography to support the conquests of the philosophic mind.

The great names repeated admiringly by every voice are those that least need our eulogies; they hold a place in the history of the sciences. But, independent of the genius who watches over scientific progress and causes it to move forward, do we not owe a debt of gratitude to those hard-working men who are concerned with details and without whose activities the [scientific] edifice would never be built? According to certain critics, the academies are too free with their eulogies. Even if this reproach is to some degree founded, should we not find it easy to pardon such an excess, which the academies will never carry far enough to excess to compensate for the jealousy and maliciousness of which the men who cultivate the sciences and letters are only too often the tools or the victims?[8]

This clear-sighted text by Vicq d'Azyr clarifies the ambiguities surrounding a disputed literary genre and assigns it a militant function. After the initial antiphrase—it is obvious that geniuses will receive more praise than ordinary men—he set forth a conception of the eulogy that is both historical and sociological, for without denying that eulogistic rhetoric was being carried to extremes in the provinces, just as Parisian philosophes were saying, he was ready to admit that eulogies were a necessity for the entire medical and scholarly elite, whose regrouping he was attempting to coordinate. In order to break the isolation of physicians and scholars, in order to have information circulated between Paris and the provinces, the merits of emulation had to be repeated untiringly; the usefulness of routine activities had to be proclaimed and justified by comparing them with great examples. There had to be instruction if there was to be motivation. Like the Parisian philosophes, Vicq d'Azyr gave preference to the historical and moral lesson; but since he was responsible before the provincial medical community, he was obliged to take into account their sensitiveness about equality and not lose sight of the apologetic role of the eulogies. This is why, in practice, he perfected a middle path within the genre, by on the one hand reserving for geniuses and noted scholars—to whom such Parisian "protectors"* and supporters as Vergennes and Watelet can be added—the long, eulogistic cadences of rhetoric in public sessions and on the other hand summarizing in brief notices the lives and work of modest physicians.

These colleagues did not become illustrious as a result of unusual inventions or immortal works; and so we do not eulogize them. It is less their names than their devotion and virtues that must be made known; and it is not for posterity but for our fellow citizens and for ourselves that we shall paint their portraits. . . . [And to conclude,] the public is not in a position to judge whether these tireless men deserved mention in our history. Severe critics say we bestow too much praise. They are right, if they are referring to the tedious self-satisfaction with which we greet everything that certain people do, write, announce, or think. They are right, if they are referring to that vile trade in eulogies in which self-interested individuals participate and to which they are attracted on all sides. In these cases, and in many others, we doubtlessly praise excessively. But when it is a matter of the modest and hard-working writer whose flagging zeal needs rekindling, or the scientific observer who devotes himself to useful research, far from those powerful individuals who distribute gold and fame, they, I say, are not sufficiently praised. I say it as an individual, and the Société Royale joins me in saying it, when it sees, scattered throughout the provinces, able physicians and surgeons who devote their evening hours to the society, without knowing whether anyone will take note of their work and even without asking for recognition, who live and die for their country, believing they are merely doing their duty, and who have no idea that any record of their great sacrifice will survive them. I say, we do not praise sufficiently, and we could never praise excessively, this sort of heroism unknown in our capital cities, where it is only fair at the least to pay homage to this heroism if we lack the strength to imitate it.[9]

And so, without admitting to the need for hyperbolic praise, Vicq d'Azyr accepted the idea of measure and fair praise for all scientists mobilized in one and the same battle. It was a requirement if they were to keep talented people bound together and make them aware that an individual's merit was decided collectively. Certainly, in practice, eulogies and notices represent a hierarchy of values and create an inequality in scholarly contributions, but this discrimination is only the reflection of recognized servitudes within the bosom of an organization that was ruled by its own norms and was fundamentally egalitarian from a social point of view.[10] In this way, listeners and readers (one might

*Each French academy has an official "protector," generally a minister or the monarch himself. This protector watched out for the interests of the academy and supplied some of the funds needed for its activities. In return he was usually consulted about the election of new members and other academic affairs.—Trans.

almost dare to write militants and sympathizers) could identify totally with the norm proposed by the society, a norm that they in turn were prepared to perpetuate and transmit. Like all academicians, they placed maximum value on a system that they personally would keep alive.[11] The eulogy, as Vicq d'Azyr envisaged it, provided models; it must be dedicated to discovering the "true principle of behavior" that formed the nucleus of each biography.[12] Every physician, every scholar admitted to the inner circle of the Société Royale—elected in the full meaning of the term, heir in the noble sense of the word, for their election constituted a succession*—of necessity had to conform to the norm. After his death, his life became a *topos*. And so, medical hagiography spread out the fan of the social virtues that it valued, proposed a list of average capacities, and brought the obscure and the genius together in an *academica mediocritas*. And even more, each speech presented living portraits within one great family, in which the use of the superlative and the constant linkage of the greatest with the very average permitted the normal and the average to be sublimated. Using social symbols to carry out its pedagogical purpose, the medical eulogy, like any other academic eulogy, idealized objective facts. Yet it presupposed precise information and documentation, which Vicq d'Azyr carefully collected. This is evident from the files of his correspondence and from allusions in the text or explicit remarks in the footnotes to his speeches. In painting a convincing and useful portrait, the secretary of the Société Royale used the time-honored canvas woven of life and work, the man and his deeds.[13] But hearing and reading Vicq d'Azyr's speeches also meant seeing him at work, here accumulating evidence,[14] there corresponding with the family, friends, and students of the deceased,[15] at another point noting and criticizing previously published eulogies,[16] and finally using the autobiography written by the dead man[17] or evoking his personal knowledge with sensitivity.[18] Beyond Vicq d'Azyr we must keep in mind the group of people corresponding with the society, "whose eyes are always on the watch over matters of public health in the different parts of the kingdom. . . . When death carries off one of these estimable men, we mourn him as a colleague who was dear to us owing to his link to the society, who was precious to us owing to his work, and whose loss leaves in our records a void that almost always is difficult to fill."[19] For the medical elite during the years preceding the Revolution, the eulogies of Vicq d'Azyr constituted the recent history of the progress of the Enlightenment. This elite could contemplate itself as it wished to see itself, involved in a tranquil heroism that was accessible to the greatest possible number. Influenced by reason, the physicians of the Société Royale pleaded the cause of talent through exemplary lives that had shown a sincerity akin to the ultimate sacrifice. In this way they collaborated in instructing citizens and arousing emulation among men of science.[20]

*Upon a member's death, a new member is elected to succeed to the empty chair. Indeed, the members of the oldest academy, the French Academy (founded in 1635), are called the "Forty Immortals" and represent the latest links in the chain of intellectual heirs descending from the original forty members. —Trans.

The medical eulogy was first of all a biography. It conferred special value upon a manner of promoting culture that the Académie de Médecine had in a way tested and accepted. But Vicq d'Azyr placed greater emphasis upon the intellectual vicissitudes than on the social foundations involved in taking the path that destiny assigns to each individual. Partially breaking away from the academic tradition of his century, although he did not neglect to evoke family origins, he was not excessively precise and showed none of the ostentatious self-satisfaction usually evident in perpetual secretaries, who were always ready to chant the genealogical litany of proofs of nobility, honors, and offices. In all, twenty-eight eulogies mention merely the father's profession, seven refer to two generations, nine (half of them are foreign associate members such as Pringle and Haller) evoke even earlier generations and sometimes mention membership in a hereditary nobility, and approximately ten provide no information at all on this matter.[21] This moderation, which is unusual in a milieu where longstanding honorable status dominated any social description, shows an optimistic view of social ascent through talent and emphasizes the cohesiveness of medical circles, since 50 percent of the eulogies involve sons, grandsons, and great-grandsons of physicians. Take the case of Hugues Maret: "Surgery having been practiced for over a century in his family, it was natural for him to study this branch of our art first of all. . . ." As the son of the surgeon major in the general hospital of Dijon, his future was in a sense guaranteed by the family's tradition as surgeons.[22] Transmission of social privileges through heredity gave way to the claim that one could rise socially as a result of talent that had been stimulated by examples within the family, for any promotion required a minimum amount of capital, an inheritance, even if only in the form of acquired behavior and virtues.

And so sons were worth what their fathers were worth. In almost two-thirds of the eulogies they are shown to have followed in their fathers' footsteps. Here we see the birth of veritable medical dynasties, but these dynasties were not formed in order to lay claim to the creation of an aristocracy based upon knowledge and merit. "When one's ancestors are so praiseworthy, can one not follow in their footsteps along the paths of study and virtue?," asked Vicq d'Azyr in the eulogy for Clément Hecquet, son and grandson of "famous physicians" and a nephew of a dean of the faculty of medicine of Paris. A man was judged by his works; the value of his life was determined by the results he achieved. It was up to each in turn to deserve the "esteem" and "public trust" that could form a part of the patrimony of men like Hecquet.[23] At the end of his career, the scholar or prestigious physician could gain a place in the nobility, but this ennoblement merely recognized his fame. Power crowned knowledge. "You may be surprised," exclaimed Vicq d'Azyr in the eulogy for Linnaeus, "that we did not announce the name of the scholar who is the subject of this eulogy as 'chevalier von Linné,' but being forced to choose between two names, one of them famous in the scientific world, the other conferred as a result of favor, we preferred the former."[24] "Select the best" was the categorical rule for social change. In the academic world of the closing years of the Ancien Régime, the physicians in the Société Royale did not so much propose bringing together the established social orders as express the largely egalitarian hopes that one could rise as a result of one's culture. And so we see why Vicq d'Azyr could criticize Hugues Maret and the members of the academy of Dijon for not having understood the importance of Jean-Jacques Rousseau's first and second academic speeches.* "How well he paints the picture of the banditry of opulence, the pride and emptiness of knowledge; how carefully he strips man of everything he considers foreign to his nature and arrays him in innocence and goodness; and how eager we are to draw near to his heart at the very moment when we stray furthest from his mind."[25] The innovative rejuvenation of the medical ethic was in part inspired by Rousseauian sensitivity.

But in actual fact, personal qualities and education formed a basis for separation and selection. Here again, however, Vicq d'Azyr brought a fortunate innovation to standard academic traditions. He spoke far less of personal qualities than of education, which always formed an essential part of the medical biography. A man's talents and favorable inclinations are indicated in less than ten eulogies,[26] and in a rather conventional way at that. A healthy and upright judgment, a good memory, tenacity toward the task at hand, or zeal for studies, and, more commonly, unflagging curiosity, were even more important than the love of truth. Truth was the attribute of both the most modest physicians, such as Jean Bouillet, the friend of Dortous de Mairan,[27] and the greatest, such as Haller.[28] Following Hunter's example, the physician could promote freedom of thought, for his profession was different from the traditional liberal professions in law or government and permitted him to *doubt* and seek the truth.[29] The medical elite wanted to be made up of astute minds and philosophes.[30]

But rather than intellectual gifts, it was education that made good physicians. We can understand why references were made to school curricula in three-fourths of the eulogies, more or less hastily, but with numerous details in the case of first-rate scholars. The absence of comments on the subject may mean that information is lacking (there are thirty-six references to *collèges* [secondary schools] or educational institutions teaching the humanities compared with forty-six references to the universities attended) or that everyone did not necessarily attend a *collège*, as was the case for apothecaries and also a few practitioners with modest social origins such as surgeons or village physicians. Only a more detailed study, which is now under way, could reveal the true importance of exceptions in this regard.

The elementary education of a physician was taken as a matter of course and was referred to without critical comment or prolonged praise. Such

*In 1749 Rousseau won a prize offered by the academy of Dijon with his "Discours sur les arts et sciences," an essay on the effects of progress and civilization upon morals. In 1752 he submitted a discourse on the "origin of inequality," but this time the academy did not award him the prize. —Trans.

training was usual and necessary, for it provided instruction in the use of Latin, which remained an essential skill for the physician of the Enlightenment. The deceased's fine Latin style in his speeches and his reading of the classics were evoked too frequently not to indicate a persisting practice.[31] On the other hand, Vicq d'Azyr dwelled upon the case of Charles Guillaume Scheele, apothecary and chemist, whose youth did not match the usual norms: "M. Scheele was sent to the public collège, but he learned so little there that his parents withdrew him to have him trained in a trade. M. Bauche, apothecary at Gotheborg, who was an old friend of the family's, offered to take him on and teach him pharmacy." And so the fourteen-year-old chemist followed the normal channels for entering a trade; but further on, Vicq d'Azyr observed, "M. Scheele doubtlessly was possessed of more than wit; but he lacked that basic education that regulates the progress of the mind and hastens its maturing. His daily work having separated him from all instruction, it must have been difficult for him to make progress, because he could learn only from books."[32] The exception confirms the rule. The members of the Société Royale, and those listening to Vicq d'Azyr, saw themselves as the *heirs* to the indispensable culture taught in collèges specializing in the humanities, without which one could not be fully a part of the scholarly elite. Yet, all education represents a choice, the disclosure of a vocation.

Young Scheele's case was a negative example of how the collège revealed the personal qualities of the future physician,[33] first of all by confirming the results obtained by education at home and then by permitting each to find his path and find it quickly. The theme of education within the family appears in half of the eulogies. It reveals the full importance of the first pedagogic steps in the development of the future elite, but it also reinforces the meaning of family traditions in transmitting knowledge and actions by visual example and by word of mouth. Happy, then, was the lad who basked in an enriching cultural atmosphere where the father, and less frequently the mother (Vicq d'Azyr's choice of words in the main stressed the role of the family as a whole), and sometimes an uncle, guided his first intellectual gropings.

M. Lorry had the good fortune to be raised in a family that was interested in fine arts, letters, and philosophy equally. His father had published a work on Justinian's *Institutes.* His elder brother took up the same career brilliantly and likewise won distinction by his writings. . . . Let us congratulate the child who is born amidst the muses and whose eyes, upon opening to the light, are struck by the models of perfection and good taste.[34]

Thus, one became culturally privileged in the cradle, and all subsequent schooling would only perfect what had already been acquired.[35] Moreover, the theme of the vocation proved that one always succeeded as a result of the patrimony he had inherited and the intellectual, moral, and social qualities he possessed. Almost half of the eulogies allude to this directly or indirectly. Take the case of M. Serrao:

When he had finished studying the humanities, powerful individuals urged him to embrace the legal profession; but he was frightened by the great number of laws and decrees that had to be learned and the contradictory texts that had to be interpreted. Medicine seemed to him free of these hindrances; the individual practicing medicine does not encounter venerable customs that form a barrier between his duty and his reason. He always deals with nature. He is always following nature's laws, and when he stops understanding, he can always stop acting.[36]

A vocation in medicine already was a touchstone for innovative behavior; hence, certainly, the stress laid upon anecdotes concerning precociousness. As in most academies, the cult of the child prodigy occupied a place of honor for, combining talent and merit, it permitted more adequate proof of the charisma, the excellence, and the superiority of those who had been elected. Take Haller's case. As soon as he could write, he began to list the words he learned in alphabetical order and compiled a Greek, Hebrew, and Chaldean dictionary that he continued to use even at an advanced age. Note that his scholarly games were not futile ones serving no future purpose. At ten he was composing Latin and German poetry and poked fun at his tutor in a Latin satire. At twelve he was reading Pierre Bayle's and Louis Moreri's dictionaries and he began to organize files for an outline of the history of science. "And so the picture of his earliest years, which in ordinary men reveals only a weak fabric, in M. Haller's case reveals the first zeal of a strong and vigorous mind and the development of genius."[37] The presence in Vicq d'Azyr's eulogies of the theme of the young philosophe and the image of the scholarly childhood reveals that the medical elite remained attached to the academic stereotype justifying both the maintenance of the ruling class in its functions and access to that class through talent, which was being insistently demanded. Successful work in school and precociousness were signs of belonging to the dominant class and at the same time proof of one's abilities. In the eyes of the physicians, they also revealed that an innovative milieu had been created to counter the retrograde tenets of the medical schools.

For, despite everything, moving on to the university caused other problems. We are familiar with the struggle that pitted the new Académie de Médecine against the powerful and venerable medical faculty of the University of Paris. So we might expect Vicq d'Azyr to make a more vigorous denunciation of medical scholasticism than he did. But in actual fact, he took a very clever position. He attacked indirectly, for he doubtlessly could not start a quarrel that, when all was said and done, the Société Royale would be sure to win, supported as it was by the central administration and by the Académie des Sciences. In addition, he may not have wanted to alienate the professors and provincial medical schools who as a group had supported the innovating movement.[38] Teachers were important supporters—note that almost half the physicians who merited a eulogy had served as professors—and it was all the more necessary to manipulate them and win them over since they held in their hands the keys to the future transformation of the scientific climate and the diffusion of the new medical norms. Vicq d'Azyr used three guidelines when evoking the reform needed in medical studies and outlining the major points of a program: describe the innovative climate in the great European universities; praise the pluralism of scholarly institutions and the resultant pedagogical eclecticism; and finally, show the importance of men, of teachers who know how to discern talent, who are encouraging and supportive, and who are the real models for reformed medicine.

Spontaneously cosmopolitan, like all the great academies, the Société Royale had international repercussions through its affiliation with associate members and correspondents residing in foreign countries. Eulogizing men elected from the cream of the scientific world made it easy to evoke the considerable advance of foreign universities over French ones. Vicq d'Azyr's major argument was that abroad a routine association existed between the teaching of medical questions and physical sciences. In his eulogy of Linnaeus, and again in his homage to Bergmann and Scheele, he had in mind the University of Uppsala. In the eulogy of Haller, teaching at Hallen, Tübingen, and especially Leyden and Basel served as the leitmotif for the pedagogical wanderings of the young scholar. The essential point for Vicq d'Azyr was that a man be confronted by multiple experiences in order to choose his path. Upon leaving the secondary school of Vexio in Smolande, Linnaeus went to Lund in Scania, where he was taken in by Stobaeus, a physician, botanist, and antiquarian. A year later he went to Uppsala, where he became the student of Olaus Celtius and of the botanist Rudbeck and taught his first classes. In 1735 he moved from one university to another in Germany, the Austrian Netherlands, and Holland. He earned a doctorate at Harderowic, spent some time in Amsterdam, and discovered in Leyden the promised land for a naturalist and physician. There he wrote his first treatises. After three studious years, he appeared in Paris, where he had his famous meeting with Bernard de Jussieu. That same year, 1738, he went to England for the first time. Back in Sweden, he practiced medicine and began to teach after a decade of travel.[39]

This was the model, the ideal: break down the barriers between institutions, broaden one's horizons, move through the fields of scholarship in order to accumulate an incalculable body of experience from the most famous teachers, where ordinary knowledge can be transformed. The institutional framework within which the change took place was of little consequence; what counted was that one could take advantage of a climate in which innovation was perceptible. Vicq d'Azyr did not a priori theorize that pedagogical progress occurred in marginal institutions; innovation could occur wherever innovators existed. MacBride, a student at Glasgow, chose his future profession near his relative, Mr. Beere, in London; then, after a training period as a surgeon on a man of war, he took courses from Smellick, professor of anatomy at the University of Dublin.[40] Charles Le Roy, with doctorates from the universities of Montpellier and Paris, studied first with Le Monnier, who was teaching physics at the Collège d'Harcourt in Paris. As a student at the University of Montpellier, he delayed reception of his doctorate in order to travel through Italy and meet the best teachers there. After having taught for twenty years, he preferred, before practicing medicine in Paris, to defend a new doctoral thesis, "convinced that a physician can offer too many proofs of his devotion to this illustrious company."[41] The great physicians remained students as long as necessary; they knew how to remain unattached. To the amphitheaters and laboratories of the Collège Royal, the greenhouses of the royal garden, the sessions of the various academies, and private laboratories such as Réamur's and Geoffroy's were available to them one after the other.[42] Paris was somewhat special in this respect compared with the other European universities, for the Parisian teachers excelled at teaching privately:

Their sound ideas, their clear and well-chosen way of expressing themselves, and the method in which they present information are indeed the qualities that characterize the lessons and work of our great teachers. That desire to please for which our nation has so often been criticized . . . has with good fortune been applied to the sciences themselves; and nowhere is the manner of making them agreeable and easy understood as it is in this capital; private courses are always to be recommended. The instruction found there is based solely on observation. One attends these classes in order to study the science of facts. The professor is stripped of all the extraneous apparatuses of the art he is teaching, and he becomes naught but a man with experience and reason. One dares to question him, even contradict him; in a word, he is superior only in his knowledge, a superiority admitted by the listeners who have freely chosen him.[43]

In this fine testimony in which his own experiences show through, Vicq d'Azyr indirectly criticized the ceremoniousness of the university courses and praised specialized lectures. He showed how the teacher-student relationship was essential to the transmission of knowledge. But the teacher was judged by his students, by their number, by their scientific merit, and by the quality of the personal relationships that were established between teacher and student. If a winner had to be declared, Boerhaave would uncontestedly have won first prize. The eulogy for his student, Jérôme Gaubius, and for van Doevren, a student of his students,[44] provided an opportunity to magnify Boerhaave's prestige and paint the portrait of a model professor:

M. Boerhaave at that time was known throughout Europe. The school at Leyden where he taught had become a school for foreigners from all nations. M. Gaubius was extremely desirous of being admitted to the school. His family having consented, he went there at once. In a crowd that presses about a great man it is easy to distinguish those who are offering their talents to an enlightened man from those who are ignorant and flatterers and who surround him as if he were an exotic creature. . . . Boerhaave took note of Gaubius. He enjoyed speaking with him, giving him personal explanations. He doubtlessly watched with pleasure those qualities developing in his disciple that would one day place him among the first rank.[45]

Though they did not win prestige comparable to Boerhaave's, many associate members—such as Barbeu-Dubourg, Spielmann, Bucquet, Loebstein, Lamurre, and Le Roy—were praised in their eulogies for having demonstrated similar professorial behavior. Though not unmindful of literary style, Vicq d'Azyr placed such emphasis upon detail in assembling his portrait gallery of great professors that we can see the importance given at the time to the role that personalities in the medical and scientific world of the universities could play as potential realizers of a transformation in education. The eulogy of the professor, the holder of a teaching chair, reveals a rough sketch of an educational reform.

Three general principles guided Vicq d'Azyr: unite those professions devoted to public health, proclaim the alliance between science and modern medicine, and articulate theoretical teachings and hospital procedures. On several occasions he denounced longstanding adversaries, old quarrels between surgeons and physicians. At the end of the eighteenth century a great distance separated the traditional barber from the surgeon, who was master of his deeds and methods. For members of the Société Royale, the hour had come to recognize this fact fully, as an element of a medical corps that was being renovated as a result of the creations of the society, which was to combine the study of internal medicine with surgical training. Therefore, in Vicq d'Azyr's opinion, Barbeu-Dubourg was wrong when he defended the medical school against the college of surgeons.[46] "Fortunately, this discussion and all the memoranda to which it gave rise have been forgotten by the impartial and judicious public, which is always able to distinguish the interests of the scholar from those of science." On the other hand, Maret, Bocquet, Lobstein, and Rose were praised for having recognized that the two disciplines complemented one another and for having promoted the study of both.[47]

Vicq d'Azyr's second reforming position had great repercussions. Without repudiating any of the principles of ancient medicine—for the airists of the Société Royale were only too aware of their debt to Galen and Hippocrates[48] —on numerous occasions he stressed the need to study the natural sciences.[49] Erudition and familiarity with authors were still praiseworthy, but above all it was important to practice scientific medicine, *Baconian* medicine in a sense. The reformed physician had to be a physicist, a chemist, and a botanist. His field should be all of nature. His method could no longer be deductive but had to be based upon scientific experiments and observation. Quackery had kept medicine in its infancy for too long. A child of time, medicine henceforth had to see itself as a child of reason.[50] Instead of learned research or systematic speculations, the professors of the medical schools should prefer the analytical study of illnesses and should propose coursework in scientific experiments, dissections, or chemical analyses that their students should be required to complete and the results of which would be discussed in their theses. But this meant that each medical faculty would require two laboratories (one for chemistry, another for anatomy), a botanical garden, and above all a hospital.[51]

Vicq d'Azyr saw teaching within a hospital setting as the only way to create a scientific approach to medicine.[52] His medicine was based on experience, on *observation,* for it explicitly required the creation of the clinic. By presenting as examples for the educated public all those who combined teaching in a medical school with training in a hospital, he was preparing the radical transformation of medical thought that Michel Foucault has traced for us.[53] Fifty years before Bichat and the changes brought by the Revolution, the clinic already existed as the creation of isolated innovators, of model practitioners, who—on occasion benefiting from government support—tended to draw generalizations on the basis of still too limited experiments in such centers as Vienna, Florence, Leyden, Edinburgh, Glasgow, or London. These attempts undoubtedly were decisive steps in preparing the institutional upheavals and theoretical developments of the future. The experience acquired at the bedsides of the hospitalized sick was, at any rate, of capital importance for a new conception of medicine:

Indeed, it is only in shelters for the poor, where wise administrators lavish help on the poor and suffering, that young physicians and surgeons can learn useful lessons. It is there, among the dying, the ill, and the convalescent, that they learn to recognize the various nuances of life and the very horrors of death. It is there that nature appears in all the disfunctions permitted by our fragile constitution. It is there that they can seek without hindrance the causes of illness in the various organs and that the student's uncertain hand can be tested on inanimate bodies. It is there that the surgeon becomes accustomed to sacrificing some part of the sensitivity that, if it exists unabated, makes him timid and trembling and, if it is entirely eliminated, changes him into a hard and even cruel man. Last, it is there that one learns to read the eyes, the features, the gestures, and the bearing of the sick and to discern those signs that the scholar notes but cannot put down in words, that one seeks in vain in books, and about which it is so important not to be mistaken.[54]

This admirable text, expressed in the compassionate rhetoric of the day, betrays a profound feeling of a new perception of the sick and of illness and issues a call for transforming practitioners through lessons in pathological anatomy and physiology.[55] Even death can teach useful lessons. Practice can teach theory, and vice versa.[56]

Talent and knowledge acquired by education could henceforth be put into concrete form in written works. I shall not summarize Vicq d'Azyr's meticulous analyses of books, when he speaks as a historian of science. The progress of discoveries, honors, and books, and their repercussions, are carefully marked out. Physicians henceforth endorsed the common position of the Enlightenment, but it is important to note where they differ from and where they resemble the scholarly elite made up of scientific enthusiasts and specialists.

Their action places them in a sphere encompassed by places and institutions. Chief among the traditional characteristics of a physician was his membership in scholarly societies; some forty of the men being praised belonged to academies and literary assemblies and, by means of competitions and meetings, found themselves totally involved in the diffusion of scientific innovations.[57] Special mention should be made of the founders of academies, such as Hugues Maret, whose work with the academy of Dijon was studied in detail. A second trait stressed in the eulogies was the need to travel and to correspond with other scholars, both very effective ways to bring about geographic integration and break down cultural barriers.[58] By this means the scholar's daily life continued the experiences he had gained during his adolescent years of study and reinforced the results of active teaching. Travel taught tolerance and multiplied one's acquaintances, and correspondence strengthened the cohesion within scholarly milieus and expanded the outlook of the European medical world to the limits of the known universe.

Take the cases of Mr. Fothergill, who received correspondence "from the most able physicians and surgeons of England,"[59] or Gaubius, who kept up a regular correspondence between Leyden and Batavia and continually exhorted "physicians and surgeons who were leaving for the Indies to obtain information about the remedies that were used there most commonly and longest."[60] And the most memorable time of Barbeu-Dubourg's life was the period during which he corresponded with Benjamin Franklin and could boast of being America's first ally in France.[61]

But the true originality of medical circles is evident in the descriptions of the places where their daily activities were usually conducted. These activities had two dimensions. One was external and, in a certain sense, collective; the other was internal, private, withdrawn. In the former, the physician was active; in the latter he reflected, meditated, wrote, and deduced some sort of lessons from previous experience. In this symmetry, this dichotomy—which is too harmonious not to betray that Vicq d'Azyr was seeking a dramatic effect—we see the two appealing types of work that we have already noted in the analysis of medical studies and that were disturbing physicians: action versus reflection, in other words, firsthand observation versus theory. Action in a hospital was the high point of the profession, the daily horizon of most members. While it was arousing fear and pity with its unpleasantness, its masses of anonymous sick, and its polluted air so like that in prisons (another place where the airists could experiment), the hospital crystallized problems and set physicians to work on them.[62] Vicq d'Azyr's emphasis upon this point—more than half the eulogies refer to it—highlights the basic cleavages between medicine for the poor and medicine for the rich, between urban and rural medical practice.

By contrast, how restful and protected were the usual retreats created by a sizable number of physicians: the botanical garden, the site of productive teaching sessions and of serene leisure in a rustic utopia of unfailing charm and almost always created to combat the unhealthy sanitary and moral influences of the big city;[63] the library and the study with their piles of books, instruments, curiosities, and specimens;[64] or the laboratory, where the scholar was reborn through the excitement of audacious experiments![65] There true liberty was unfurled in silence, without constraint, and was not disturbed by the questions of a small number of students who were permitted to cross the threshold and enter the hideaway. While spending several years in the library of Cyrillo, his teacher, the Neapolitan Serrao imagined he saw there "a host of great men by whom he felt surrounded and whom his imagination pictured as ready to transmit to him their knowledge. His eyes would fill with tears. He would pass rapidly through the gallery. His impatient hands would touch everything, yet continue on. He would have liked to learn everything, comprehend everything in an instant." Cyrillo entered in the midst of this ecstacy: "'Oh, Master,' cried the young man, dashing up to him. 'I am happy for you, for in putting me at the source of Enlightenment, you have unveiled to me the past, and I am answerable to you for it in the future!'"[66]

In this little word-picture, which bears such a close resemblance to one of Greuze's painting, Vicq d'Azyr focused on one of the main lessons taught by the eulogies: the correct use of science involved a choice between the happiness of a scholarly retreat and the difficulties of medical practice. He was urging innovative physicians to make a commitment, a true political act. To lead them to this decision, he proposed goals and means to achieve them, he informed them of the steps to be taken and the personal qualities that were indispensable if they were to succeed.

First off, he focused on their conduct. The medical eulogies provide a list of exemplary behavior where everything is related to a moralized action. There are two separate categories of virtues—those of the private man and those of the public man—that are common to all the academic eulogies, and these virtues paint pictures of mores that exemplify the ideal found in the manners books of the time. As far as the former category was concerned, Vicq d'Azyr was not very original, and his physicians all have the qualities of the *sensitive* individual; they display tenderness and modesty, are fair and kind hearted, cry easily. His use of colorless adjectives and his manipulation of conventional clichés that are rarely given life by personal anecdotes make this portrait gallery a shadow show dominated by oratory. But the puppet conveying the individual's morals and character permitted Vicq d'Azyr to evoke a conflict and hence to instruct and persuade. He saw one's moral fate as less important than one's intellectual fulfillment, which provided proof of philosophical progress; but his word-picture permitted him to magnify the social role played by the physician and hence to pick out the essential traits. By contrasting calm and tranquil happiness with the civic heriosm shown by the committed practitioner, he offered his audience a medical ethic based on action and showed the men of the Enlightenment that it was important to know how to choose.

The predominant qualities were those of a wise stoic: equability, orderliness, only occasional severity, well-balanced and controlled emotions, and healthy and temperate living. A training period for action took shape in the calm of an untroubled family life, in the tranquillity of a quiet and agreeable existence, where warm friendship counted for a great deal. This picture of the hideaway, shut off from the world, served all the more to prove the merits of the sacrifice made by the individual who knew how to answer duty's call.[67] In the same fashion, wealth was sure to reward outstanding merit.[68] An adequate but average income was the lot of the great majority[69] and made it possible for them to be independent;[70] greater material success merely confirmed greater devotion and was only acceptable and justifiable when the money went for useful projects, when it made philanthropy possible. The moral position of the medical profession could only be one of service.

Into the academic world, where the idea of a behavior socialized by culture was triumphant—*Vir amabilis ad societatem*—Vicq d'Azyr introduced the idea of submission to patriotic duty. In order to do so, the physician had to appear as his true self. His appearance, his gestures, and his words had to correspond to his benevolent mission. Three qualities were required of the physician. *Prima est scientia,* and we have seen how the reform in studies and scientific undertakings met this need; *secunda facundia,* that is, smooth elocution, the ability to express oneself well; and *tertia comitas,*[71] in other words, affability, a benevolent manner. So we can see why Lieutaud was hesitant about his vocation: "He was afraid that his misshapen body and cold disposition would prove an obstacle to success in the practice of medicine. He could have spared himself this anxiety, had he reflected that in order to win public confidence it is less a question of pleasing than of paying attention and that he who treats the public more firmly is not always he who receives the least number of caresses from it."[72]

The spoken word and physical appearances were essential in one's medical connections. Robust health permitted the physician to face the fatigue of the profession; an affable and gentle manner permitted him to be more persuasive. Let us see how Lorry conducted himself:

A profound study of his art made him truly worthy of his success and his moral qualities won him the friendship of all those who summoned him; humane and compassionate, he had no difficulty in pleasing. In order to appear affable, he did not need to study his gestures, control the posture of his healthy body, mute the timbre of his voice, bank the fire of his thoughts, or conceal the impulses of his strong will. Nature had made him affable; that is, by giving him wit, finesse, and gaity, it had also given him sensitivity, the gentleness without which the mind is almost always unwieldy for those who use it and dangerous for those against whom it is aimed. His agreeability was shown in his manners, in his speech, and in his advice. When working with the sick, it was his chief tool and it decreased their distaste of all the other tools, tempered the severity of their treatment, went to their very souls, and calmed them by making these souls stronger and less heedful of pain.[73]

This description, which doubtlessly used old clichés, shows clearly the desire to promote a view that illness could be conquered, could be decreased or weakened when confronted by the power of language and the virtues of sociability. Vicq d'Azyr demonstrated a basic optimism that tried to exorcize the old collective misfortunes and made it possible to advance without fear to the frontiers of extreme distress.

It remains to define the principles of a reasoned activity. Vicq d'Azyr proposed two particularly effective ones. First, the struggle against charlatanism, "a kind of monster about which everyone in general laments but which everyone in particular welcomes."[74] And second, the establishment of a veritable medicine for the masses. In the first case, he was inspired by one of the goals of the thinkers of the Enlightenment: "From the abuses committed in the name of religion, medicine, and astronomy, three great sources of evil arose: fanaticism, charlatanism, and superstition."[75] The battle fought by the medical profession pitted reason against prejudice. Its importance stems from the fact that it took the actual situation into account; for, indeed, most rural people still never consulted physicians and in their poverty and misfortune could only obtain the care of healers and charlatans of all sorts. Vicq d'Azyr held that the charlatans succeeded owing to the ignorance of the masses. Their "miracles" could not succeed before enlightened viewers.[76] Confronted by "aberrations of the mind," the innovating physician had to reveal the origins, causes, and dangers of such aberrations. He was the judge in the court of reason, a missionary for the propagation of the Enlightenment. This was true for Serrao, who was able to convince the elite of Naples about the deceptions involved in tarantism.[77] It was also true for Girod:

Travelling incessantly within his province, where public trust followed him continually, he took advantage of this opportunity to enlighten the people about their basic needs. He fought prejudice and exterminated error; his approach put to flight those clumsy charlatans who, lacking sufficient wit to fool city dwellers, invade the countryside and sell hope and poison to the credulous farm worker.[78]

Doubtlessly insensitive to the degree to which prejudices were rooted in popular culture, the innovating physicians of the Société Royale attacked the miraculous, the world of the imaginary. Their reverence for skepticism and for freedom of thought presupposed a triumphant scientism justified by the idea of collective service. They were "physicians of the poor," "benefactors of the indigent,"[79] servants of the "public good." And so the eulogy developed into a program. The mobilization of the total energy within the medical professions was, as Jean Meyer has shown, strictly utilitarian.[80] On many occasions Vicq d'Azyr detailed the agenda for a fight that was just beginning. He described the outposts, depicted the weapons. The reformed physician would serve the humble; benevolence, through charity organized by laymen within society, was the physician's essential virtue and would guide him to avoid all ostentatious behavior. "How, indeed, could the common people, who were not very accustomed to finding the rich compassionate, dare to describe their infirmities to someone who seemed to lofty to descend to their level and attend to their suffering?"[81]

The physician's battlefield was the epidemic. The expression *médecin des épidémies* appears in almost half the texts. In some cases, such as the eulogy for Vétillard,[82] Vicq d'Azyr was satisfied to enumerate the long list of epidemic illnesses that were cared for by the physician he was honoring. For the most humble and the most famous, it was the true battle ground:

Independently of the causes affecting each individual's health, there are general causes whose influence extends to all the inhabitants of a region, where they spread illnesses of one and the same sort, the source of which is often hidden, the exact nature doubtful, and the treatment uncertain. He who proposes providing useful care under distressing circumstances must combine knowledge with prudence and firmness. It is not enough to possess the information required by the everyday practice of our art. In the quality of the air and water, the nature of the foods eaten, and the climate, and through the scrupulous study of everything that went before, he must be capable of finding the cause of the illness he wants to stop from spreading. He must go back to its very first appearance, follow its path, find out how it was spread, and limit the contagion (once he has determined that it exists). He must, in a sense, rise above the humanity to whose succor he is hastening, and, having disregarded all the dangers surrounding him, he must reassure, console, and bring calm wherever he goes, while at the same time bringing back good health.[83]

In this eulogy for Navier, we can see the inquiries that Vicq d'Azyr was proposing to the medical elite of his day. Engaged in a vast, collective undertaking, this elite almost always received government help. Here medical despotism and enlightened absolutism joined forces in charitable work that involved both welfare and correction. The indispensable qualities of the physician were those necessary to individuals "who have men to govern and to lead."[84] Providing care meant administering.

The eulogy of Lieutaud is a good example of this conception, which saw talent as lodged in the governing class. Science would languish without government protection. The eulogies for several foreign physicians—Tozetti and Sanchez, for example—provided an occasion to demonstrate the benefits of the alliance between the medical profession and those in power. Spread through the provinces, *officiers de santé* [health officers] (note the choice of words and think of the old connotations of the office and the future in store for it) should enjoy the honors and prerogatives related to their work, they should benefit from the reward due their service, "in a word, it is in their interest to form but one great body whose soul should be honor and love of work."[85] *Patriote, citoyen utile* [patriot, useful citizen],[86] the physician of the Société Royale de Médecine bore witness to the merit-based elite's demand to attain the rank they believed their due. They also show how the support of the monarchical state could still divert this elite from a clearer awareness of their future. In Vicq d'Azyr's eulogies we glimpse the full strength of a collective idea mobilized for the reforms that led to revolutions. Perhaps part of the strength of this idea also derived from the degree to which it proposed a picture of the physician as a man with knowledge and reason, as a missionary for a sacred cause but not a fanatic, vindicated by his devotion and sacrifice.

The apotheosis of the eulogy, the deaths of these physicians bring to mind (not without intentional irony) the unreliability of medicine. Here the Société Royale was following the tendencies of the academies, that is, establishing the secular veneration of great men and transforming merit into recognition of immortality. In its way a collective mystique was at work, and the medical originality is clearly revealed in the definitive naturalization of an interest in the macabre and in the absence of any reference to religion (only one in fifty-four eulogies). Physicians died rationally; their passing was but an opportunity to show how the apology had been transferred from the religious to the social sphere. The deaths of physicians provided the ultimate proof of their commitment as militants. Three-fourths of their deaths were blamed directly upon the fatigue and danger of their "ministry." Almost half of them had been involved in a fatal epidemic. It was while carrying out their tasks that they proved their greatness and their heroism. Girod, from the Franche-Comté, learned that an epidemic had broken out and hurried to the spot; stricken in turn, he realized from the symptoms that he would not survive. "He announced this and he died."[87] Maret, from the province of Burgundy, died a victim of his own zealousness. He set out for Fresne-Saint-Mamès, where an epidemic of fever had broken out. No sooner had he arrived than he too fell ill, but he continued to carry on his work. "He was a contagious sick man who visited the other sick and tried to bring them back to the life that he himself was about to leave." While lying delirious on his pallet, he spoke only of the local victims of the epidemic. When he regained consciousness:

Perhaps at that point he realized the full extent of the sacrifice he was about to accomplish; he may also have recalled that he had been a citizen before he was a father. What other feeling than duty, what other strength than that of a noble thought, can provide support during those moments of decline and death, when one's final memories should be of the good and evil one has done.[88]

Dr. Maret's neoclassical death shows how the ceremonies in the City of Lights [Paris, also the "City of Enlightenment"] greeted a secularized apology of sacrifice.

Having reached the end of this analysis, we can view the eulogies of the Société Royale de Médecine as one of the basic tools in the social mobilization of talent and merit. Presented in order to provide examples for the history of the progress of the medical mind, during the final two decades of the Ancien Régime they served as a catalyst for a demand for equitable promotion. They were modeled after the procedures of the universities and learned societies. To realize this, one has only to reread the eulogies for Bergman and Pringle. These eulogies justified promotion by merit through a two-pronged argument: in the name of science and reason, the medical elite knows that providing care means governing and directing; it feels that it has proved its political capability by virtue of its devotion and sacrifice. When this elite claimed to be made up of patriotic physicians and citizens, it was not a hollow statement. Engaged in a collective movement that could not grow in the absence of enthusiasm, it called for a scientific reform through a change in social procedures. A spontaneously collective and administrative medicine was born without in any way violating the Hippocratic oath. A desire to provide welfare was born of this encounter. Vicq d'Azyr's eulogies mark one step in the development of modern medical ideologies and mentalities. Yet it would be completely wrong to think that these eulogies are sufficient evidence on their own. That would mean mistaking one's prey for a shadow, a reflection for reality. The questions that these eulogies raise will undoubtedly lead to other inquiries in this field, inquiries based on other sources. Moreover, the work now under way shows that we are not dealing with a pious wish.

NOTES

1. Jean Meyer, "L'Enquête de l'Académie de Médecine sur les épidémies, 1774-1794," in *Médecins, climat et épidémies à la fin du XVIIIᵉ siècle* (Paris-The Hague: Mouton, 1972), pp. 9-20; Daniel Roche, *Le Siècle des Lumières en province: Académies et académiciens provinciaux, 1680-1789* (in press).

2. J.-P. Peter, "Malades et maladies à la fin du XVIIIᵉ siècle," in *Médecins, climat, et épidémies*, p. 137.

3. Vicq d'Azyr, *Eloges des membres de la Société Royale de Médecine* (Paris, 1778); and idem., *Mémoires de la Société Royale de Médecine*, 10 vols. (Paris, 1776-89). To my knowledge the only complete series is in the library of the museum of natural history in Paris (call number Pr 661-1.10). See also F. Dubois, *Eloges lus dans les séances publiques de l'Académie Royale de Médecine* (Paris, 1859). For the still-to-be-written history of the genre, one can consult Vicq d'Azyr's manuscripts and correspondence in the archives of the Academy of Medicine, cartons 100-170; cf. Meyer, "L'Enquête de l'Académie de Médecine," pp. 9-10.

4. Archives départementales, Côte-d'Or, archives of the academy of Dijon, register 10, 27 April 1780.

5. Indeed, there are less than ten eulogies for nonphysicians: those for Etienne Mignot de Montigny, a member of the Academy of Sciences; Hervé Duhamel de Monceau, also a member of the Academy of Sciences; Claude-Henri Watelet, of the French Academy; François-Paul Poulletier de La Salle; and Charles Gravier de Vergennes. To this could be added the biographical notices about M. de Joubert, a native-born associate at Port-au-Prince [in today's Haiti],, and of chevalier Lefebvre Deshayes.

6. Vicq d'Azyr, *Mémoires*, 1:16. For background reading, cf. P. Astruc, "Eloges prononcés à la Société Royale de Médecine par Vicq d'Azyr," *Progrès médical* (1951).

7. D'Alembert, *Encyclopédie*, 5: 526-27; see also Thomas, *Essai sur les éloges* (Paris, 1773), pp. 463-67; and, for a discussion of the context, see Roche, *Le Siècle des Lumières en province*, chap. 3, "L'Homme académique."

8. Vicq d'Azyr, "Eloge de Jean-Baptiste Luc Planchon," *Mémoires*, 3: 154-55.

9. Idem, "Notice," ibid., 5: 200, 215-16; and 10: xxxvi, for 1789.

10. The average number of pages allowed for a eulogy was twenty-two and the average for notices was two and a half pages per person praised, for totals of twenty-eight and twenty-six, respectively.

11. P. Bourdieu and J.-C. Passeron, *La Reproduction* (Paris, 1970); P. Bourdieu and M. de Saint-Martin, "L'Excellence scolaire," *Annales, E.S.C.* (1970), pp. 146-75; idem, "Les Catégories de l'entendement professoral," *Actes de la recherche en sciences sociales*, no. 3 (1975), pp. 68-93.

12. Vicq d'Azyr, *Mémoires*, 6: 4, for 1787.

13. The principal items in the traditional questionnaire were: date and place of birth, name at christening and names of parents; social status and connections of the family; education and teachers; beginnings in the world, travels; tastes and subjects studied; methods used in study; bibliography of published and unpublished works; reputation; principal facts of private and public life; character, morals, health, fortune. See Roche, *Le Siècle des Lumières en province*, chap. 3, pt. 3, "L'Homme académique," esp. nn. 37, 38.

14. Vicq d'Azyr, "Eloges de Fothergill," *Mémoires*, 4: 52; "Eloge de Sanchez," ibid., 217, 237.

15. Idem, "Eloge de Sanchez," ibid., 4: 236, "Asked by us to send details . . ."; "Eloge de Lamure, ibid., 7: 168.

16. Idem, "Eloge de Bergman," ibid., 5: 141 ff.

17. Ibid., 142.

18. Idem, "Eloge de Macquer," ibid., 5: 94.

19. Ibid., 4: 168.

20. This had been the wish of philosophes ever since Fontenelle; cf. Thomas, *Essai sur les éloges*, chap. 2.

21. Conversely, of over a thousand academic eulogies analyzed for the eighteenth century, only 10 percent are silent about the individual's origins (20 percent for the Société Royale, but the low number of examples forces us to view this percentage as a mere indication). References to illustrious, old, or honorable families are found in only 20 percent of the eulogies by Vicq d'Azyr, though the average for the entire century is 40 percent. See Roche, *Le Siècle des Lumières en province*, chap. 3, pt. 3.

22. Vicq d'Azyr, "Eloge de Maret," *Mémoires,* 7: 128-65.

23. Idem, "Eloge de Hecquet," ibid., 7: 50-54 (chap. 7).

24. Idem, "Eloge de Linné," ibid., 2: 17-44; see also "Eloge de Haller," ibid., 1: 78-79.

25. Idem, "Eloge de Maret," ibid., 7: 139. An uncontestable Rousseauian echo can be found in the eulogies for Haller and Speilmann (ibid., 5: 116). Being a member of an old patrician family was at the time an indication of probity. "As early as the fourteenth century the Spielmann family was included among the patricians, but it never attempted to rise above the class of the bourgeoisie. The house that the elder Spielmann occupied, and in which he wished to see his son settle, had been passed on to him by his ancestors. In small cities where luxury is uncommon, one can still find a small number of such families that do not attempt to rise above their estate, that limit their ambitions to seeing their probity pass on to their children like an inheritance. The roof they receive from their fathers, and under which their workshops are set up, is simple, as they are, and old, like their family; and their genealogy, without stain and likewise without illustriousness, is written in the memory of the numerous people who hold them in honor. This spectacle, now very rare in our cities, is still rather common in some of those in Switzerland and Germany."

26. Roche, *Le Siècle des Lumières en province,* chap. 3, pt. 3. More than one-third of the eulogies analyzed refer to the intellectual qualities shared by academicians.

27. Daniel Roche, "Un Savant et sa bibliothèque au XVIIIe siècle: Les Livres de J.-J. Dortous de Mairan, secrétaire perpétuel de l'Académie des Sciences," *Dix-huitième siècle* 1 (1969): 47-88.

28. Vicq d'Azyr, *Mémoires,* 1: 59-93.

29. Ibid., 4: 183-208.

30. Idem, "Eloge de Desmery," ibid., 5: 205-6.

31. Idem, "Eloge de Lorry," ibid., 5: 39, 53; "Eloges de Sanchez," ibid., 4: 213; "Eloge de Le Roy," ibid., 3: 48; "Eloge de Serrao," ibid., 7: 68.

32. Idem, "Eloge de Scheele," ibid., 7: 89.

33. Idem, "Eloge de Lorry," ibid., 1: 26. "The famous Rollin took pleasure in personally directing M. Lorry's studies. His success in the *collège* was among that restricted number that promises real success at a more advanced age. This success was not solely the fruit of a facile memory or persistent work; imagination and taste were the chief factors. He never forgot, and his friends often reminded him of, the following anecdote. It was a question of expressing in Latin verse the excitement of New Year's Day for a contest. . . . This scene was sketched by M. Lorry in the two lines that follow, which were deemed worthy of the prize: *Haec est illa dies qua plebs vesana fureusque se fugiendo petit, sequée petenda fugit.*"

34. Ibid., p. 25.

35. Idem, "Eloge de Le Roy," ibid., 3: 33; "Eloge de Sanchez," ibid., 4: 209; "Eloge de Pringle," ibid., 4: 183.

36. Idem, "Eloge de Serrao," ibid., 7: 67-68; See also "Eloge de Bouillet," ibid., 1: 43-44; "Eloge de Linné," ibid., 2: 18-19; "Eloge de Le Roy," ibid., 3: 34-35; "Eloge de Bucquet," ibid., 3: 75; "Eloge de Lieutaud," ibid., 3: 95; "Eloge de Gaubius," ibid., 3: 119-20; "Eloge de Planchon," ibid., 3: 148; "Eloge de Butet," ibid., 4: 172; "Eloge de Hunter," ibid., 4: 183-84; "Eloge de Sanchez," ibid., 4: 209-10; "Eloge de Macquer," ibid., 5: 69; "Eloge de Targioni," ibid., 5: 95-96; "Eloge de Cusson," ibid., 5k: 127-28; "Eloge de Bergman," ibid., 5: 141-43; "Eloge de Marrigues," ibid., 7: 54; "Eloge de Lobstein," ibid., 7: 50; "Eloge de Scheele," ibid., 7: 89-90.

37. Idem, "Eloge de Haller," ibid., 1: 60-61. For other examples see those cited in note 36, especially the eulogies of Le Roy and Lobstein.

38. Between 1776 and 1789, more than a hundred professors were among associate members and correspondents of the society. In addition it won approval from the medical faculties of Montpellier, Aix, Angers, Caen, Bourges, Douai, Nancy, Nantes, Perpignan, Poitier, Rheims, Strasbourg, and Toulouse. It was also on good terms with numerous medical "colleges," that is, professional groups that often carried out educational activities. These colleges were located in Abbeville, Amiens, Béziers, Bordeaux, Clermont-Ferrand, Dieppe, Dijon, Grenoble, La Rochelle, Le Mans, Lille, Limoges, Lyons, Marseilles, Montauban, Moulins, Nancy, Nîmes, Orléans, Rennes, Rouen, and Troyes. The importance of the cities with academies can be observed in the laurels awarded to supporters; see Roche, *Le Siècle des Lumières en province,* chap. 5: "Les Institutions de la république des lettres."

39. Vicq d'Azyr, "Eloge de Linné," *Mémoires,* 2: 18-19, 21-22, 33-34.

40. Idem, "Eloge de Mac Bride," ibid., 2: 53-55.

41. Idem, "Eloge de Le Roy," ibid., 3: 34-35, 50. See also "Eloge de Nobleville," ibid., 2: 46.

42. Idem, "Eloge de Cusson," ibid., 5: 127; "Eloge de Marrigues," ibid., 7: 54; "Eloge de Spielmann," ibid., 5: 120-22.

43. Idem, "Eloge de Gaubius," ibid., 3: 12.

44. Ibid., p. 122; "Eloge de Van Doevren," ibid., 5: 188-89.

45. Idem, "Eloge de Gaubius," ibid., 3: 123-24.

46. J. Barbeu-Dubourg, Lettre à l'abbé Desfontaines au sujet de la maîtrise ès arts (Paris, 1743); Vicq d'Azyr, "Eloge de Barbeu-Dubourg," Mémoires, 2: 64; Jean-Pierre Goubert and F. Lebrun, "Médecins et chirurgiens dans la société française du XVIIIᵉ siècle," Annales cisalpines d'histoire sociale 4 (1974): 119-36.

47. Vicq d'Azyr, "Eloge de Bucquet," Mémoires, 3: 90; "Eloge de Rose," ibid., 5: 205; "Eloge de Lobstein," ibid., 7: 59; and "Eloge de Maret," ibid., 7: 131-32.

48. Idem, "Eloge de Le Roy," ibid., 3: 39-48; "Eloge de Navier," ibid., 3: 52; "Eloge de Fothergill," ibid., 4: 53-54; "Eloge de Sanchez," ibid., 4: 209; "Eloge de Serrao," ibid., 5: 72; "Eloge de Lamure," ibid., 7: 165, 172.

49. Idem, "Eloge de Bouillet," ibid., 1: 49, 52; "Eloge de Halle," ibid., 1: 65; "Eloge de Bucquet," ibid., 3: 81; "Eloge de Lieutaud," ibid., 3: 98; "Eloge de Pringle," ibid., 4: 139; "Eloge de Lorry," ibid., 5: 32-33; "Eloge de Targioni," ibid., 5: 100; "Eloge de Bergman," ibid., 5: 148; "Eloge de Van Doevren," ibid., 5: 188; "Eloge de Maret," ibid., 7: 151-52; and "Eloge de Lamure," ibid., 7: 176.

50. Idem, "Eloge de Van Doevren," ibid., 5: 190-91.

51. Idem, "Eloge de Lamure," ibid., 7: 179-80.

52. Peter, "Malades et maladies," p. 137.

53. Michel Foucault, Naissance de la Clinique: Une Archéologie du regard médical (Paris, 1963).

54. Vicq d'Azyr, "Eloge de Mac Bride," Mémoires, 2: 54.

55. Peter, "Malades et maladies," pp. 256-57.

56. Vicq d'Azyr, "Eloge de Targioni," Mémoires, 5: 100-101.

57. Idem, "Eloge de Lorry," ibid., 5: 46.

58. Nineteen and eighteen instances, respectively. Good examples can be found in idem, "Eloge de Cusson," ibid., 5: 128-89, and "Eloge de Sanchez," ibid., 4: 213.

59. Idem, "Eloge de Fothergill," ibid., 4: 70-71.

60. Idem, "Eloge de Gaubius," ibid., 3: 133-34.

61. Idem, "Eloge de Barbeu-Dubourg," ibid., 2: 71-72.

62. Idem, "Eloge de Fothergill," ibid., 4: 55; "Eloge de Pringle," ibid., 4: 139; "Eloge de Lorry," ibid., 5: 33; "Eloge de Lieutaud," ibid., 3: 99-100.

63. Idem, "Eloge de Darluc," ibid., 5: 214-15.

64. Idem, "Eloge de Hunter," ibid., 4: 204-5 (where the description of the veritable anatomical museum set up by Hunter ends with this remark: "It was in this museum that he gave his lessons in anatomy"); "Eloge de Sanchez," ibid., 4: 225; "Eloge de Lorry," ibid., 5: 32.

65. Idem, "Eloge de Spielmann," ibid., 5: 11.

66. Idem, "Eloge de Serrao," ibid., 3: 70-71.

67. Idem, "Eloge de Fothergill," ibid., 3: 77-78.

68. Idem, "Eloge de Gaubius," ibid., 3: 141.

69. In all there are five references to sizable fortunes, evidence of the individual's great success, and ten references to average or modest wealth: idem, "Eloge de Lieutaud," ibid., 3: 116; "Eloge de Fothergill," ibid., 4: 51-52; "Eloge de Harmant," ibid., 4: 4; "Eloge de Buttet," ibid., 4: 171; "Eloge de Lorry," ibid., 5: 32, 36.

70. Idem, "Eloge de Lobstein," ibid., 7: 58.

71. Idem, "Eloge de Serrao," ibid., 7: 81.

72. Idem, "Eloge de Lieutaud," ibid., 3: 10.

73. Idem, "Eloge de Lorry," ibid., 5: 31-32.

74. Idem, "Eloge de Gaubius," ibid., 3: 133-34.

75. Idem, "Eloge de Serrao," ibid., 7: 75.

76. Idem, "Eloge de Lieutaud," ibid., 3: 114.

77. Idem, "Eloge de Serrao," ibid., 7: 76-80.

78. Idem, "Eloge de Girod," ibid., 5: 63-64. There are a total of twelve instances of the struggle against charlatanism. The theme of inoculation was comparable, with ten references. In discussing the question, Vicq d'Azyr at no point took a stand against the latter practice,

though he called for prudence and care. See especially "Eloge de Girod," ibid., 7: 148; and "Eloge de Serrao," ibid., 7: 86. On this question the eulogies reveal subtle differences from the opinion held by Jean Meyer, "L'Enquête de l'Académie de Médecine," p. 11, n. 1.

79. Twenty-six uses of the former expression, and roughly ten for the second. The word *bienfaisance* [good deeds] appears in some twenty eulogies.

80. Meyer, "L'Enquête de l'Académie de Médecine," p. 12.

81. Vicq d'Azyr, "Eloge de Bucquet," *Mémoires*, 3: 89.

82. Ibid., 4: 170-71.

83. Idem, "Eloge de Navier," ibid., 3: 55-56.

84. Idem, "Eloge de Planchon," ibid., 3: 15.

85. Idem, "Eloge de Lieutaud," ibid., 3: 111-12.

86. The two expressions appear twenty-one times. Government support was evoked in half the eulogies.

87. Vicq d'Azyr, *Mémoires*, 5: 65.

88. Ibid., 7: 160.

5
Work-Related Diseases of Artisans in Eighteenth-Century France

Arlette Farge

A body at work is a body that exerts and spends itself, accomplishing a routine sequence of gestures and movements in a specific place. In the case of the eighteenth-century workshops and artisans, one can easily imagine the harsh, precarious, and unsafe conditions in which work was accomplished. Poor health, injuries, and incurable diseases were part of the daily landscape, as common as insufficient wages, ill-ventilated workshops, and job insecurity.

About this subject the physicians of the time had relatively little to say. By comparison with the as yet underused mass of documents concerning epidemics, women's diseases, Caesarean section, or the medical topography of a specific village, books or manuscripts written with the purpose of describing work-related diseases remain rare. This very scarcity is one of the things that arouses the researcher's interest. Whenever there is a trace of a new medical subject matter, one must attempt to decode its significances, to find out whether it points to the emergence of a new sensibility or whether it had become necessary to "deal with" the matter. In reading these documents, one must find beneath or beyond the words the various areas of concern that have gone into the making of the text. One must recognize the constant interchange between the levels at which the author, whether physician or member of the enlightened elite—inspector of workshops, for instance—in his efforts to describe a situation and then to draw conclusions, made use of such varied concerns as humanitarian sentiment, profound indignation in the face of overwhelming and visible misfortune, and a need to persuade, to reconcile an interest in hygiene, morality, and health with a quasi-natural acceptance of the order of things, which included the poor man at work.

While the number of such documents is not unlimited, they are by no

Annales, E.S.C. 32 (September-October 1977): 998-1006. Translated by Elborg Forster.

means impossible to find. Everyone knows about the book by the Italian Bartolomeo Ramazzini, *Essai sur les maladies des artisans*. This work first appeared at Modena in 1700. A few years later, it was translated and published in Germany. Then, in 1713, it was reprinted once again at Padua. A French edition was published by Moutard in 1777, quite late in the century.[1]

It appears that Ramazzini was a pioneer in this field. To be sure, physicians had already had occasion to observe some diseases of artisans. Fernel, for instance, reported that a midwife, having delivered a woman afflicted with venereal disease at home, contracted a sore. In the collected papers of the various academies one finds a few observations of the same type. The *Philosophical Transactions* of the Royal Society of London of 1665, for instance, include a short paper on the miners of Fréjus.

On the other hand, the authors who dealt with the diseases of artisans in general, such as Philippe Hecquet,[2] Dr. Buchan,[3] and a few others, never did more than reiterate the various classifications and comments of Ramazzini, and their publications clearly owed everything to the Italian author. Others published more innovative work on the diseases of specific kinds of artisans, such as painter's colic or the diseases of ships' crews, but there were not many of these authors.

In the early nineteenth century, Panckoucke's *Dictionnaire des sciences médicales* was to deal at length with the diseases of artisans, either in the articles devoted to a specific disease or in the analyses of the individual crafts.[4] Under the heading "occupation," the author of the entry ended by saying that it would be some time before a complete treatise could be written. This confirms—if it needs to be confirmed—that this was indeed a new subject in the eighteenth century.

Nor do the manuscript archives of the Société Royale de Médecine[5] contain many letters or medical reports on this problem. However, I found seven documents that are of interest in this connection, all of them dating from the end of the eighteenth century. In 1780, Colombot, physician at Besançon, sent the Société the outline of a history of disease. In a few pages he discusses those of hatters and clockmakers.[6] In the same year, Beerenbrock of Montpellier contributed a short piece[7] on the diseases of gilders, while Chevandier, physician of the town of Serres in the High Alps, wrote a very short memorandum on the diseases of various artisans. More interesting because of their wealth of detail, the four memoranda by Pajot des Charmes[8] are outstanding for their precision and the richness of their data. The author was deputy inspector of workshops, not a physician. Nonetheless, he was named correspondent of the Société on the basis of his work. His perspective was that of an elite charged with fostering the harmonious development of French industry at the end of a century in which a massive preindustrialization was already perceptible. The present essay is primarily concerned with studying this perspective. Two complementary approaches will be used to apprehend the discourse of Pajot des Charmes and, through him, that of a dominant group in society looking at its country's laboring class. As a first step, I shall try to analyze how the work place and the motions involved in the various occupations, some of which inevitably condemned the worker to injury and disease, were described; as a second step, I shall use what is said and what is not said in the text to bring out an underlying set of ideologies and sensibilities.

This amounts to more than showing us, who are living in the twentieth century, the work-related diseases that were perceived in the eighteenth century. I am interested in discerning as much as possible of the consciousness of the elites at the end of the Ancien Régime who were concerned about the laboring classes, knowing that those classes were indispensable, if only to the elite's own wealth.

A Violent and Death-Dealing
Environment: The Workshop

At the time, no one would have denied the importance and necessity of studying the connections between work and disease. It was a new field, and there was a certain pride in its development: not only was it to everyone's advantage to combat the diseases of artisans, but to do so also demonstrated an honorable desire to foster the well-being of humanity. Pajot des Charmes made this point in the conclusion of his memorandum on the diseases of cloth workers:[9] "There is no doubt that it is quite possible to find ways to prevent them; consequently it would be *worthy* of the Société Royale de Médecine to offer prizes or other rewards to persons who, in their noble desire to share the humanitarian concern pervading this body of distinguished scholars, might suggest the means of banishing the evils besetting the multitudinous class." And the members of the Société who drew up its reports, well aware that Pajot des Charmes was a sensitive humanitarian, realized that his memoranda contained directly applicable ideas: "Such aspirations testify to a sensitive soul, concerned with the well-being of humanity. We feel that an abridged version of his observations should be included in the Société's report; they will be valuable materials for the history of work-related diseases that is now being assembled by the Société."[10]

In the introduction to his translation of Ramazzini's book, Fourcroy stressed "the interest of such a study in connection with the ongoing research about epidemics." A footnote reads: "It is to be wished that the Société Royale de Médecine, whose work extends to all useful areas, enjoin its corresponding physicians in the provinces to study the local artisans, especially in the context of their descriptions of epidemic conditions."

Possibly because of a positive new interest in collecting all the facts concerning the history of work-related diseases among artisans,[11] the tone employed by Pajot des Charmes and others in describing life in the workshop wavered among blitheness, straightforward reporting, and sometimes real but restrained indignation. But perhaps the restrained tone is due simply to the certainty that it was as yet impossible to mitigate the suffering that was so often called inevitable. If this was the nature of things, what could be said about it? "Are we not forced to agree that several crafts are a source of suffering to those who practice them?"[12] To agree, to write, to describe already means to admit, to recognize, to become aware. The relatively serene and always precise vocabulary used to describe sometimes insufferable working conditions, which stretched the human body beyond endurance and destroyed its health as well as its dignity, testify to the manner in which the notables "could" speak about the people. They were there to mitigate the harm, not to revolt. It was in this endeavor that they found their dignity. Only once in these long memoranda does the word "revolt" appear in connection with the glassworkers and the air they breathe: "Every stranger is revolted by the stale and mephitic odor that pervades the workshops." Does "stranger" mean foreigner or stranger to the condition of the workers? However that may be, he can be revolted because he is an outsider. Pajot des Charmes had other things to do, namely, to work for improvements or to instigate research that would solve the problem. Discretion, forthrightness, direct description based on information of a scientific nature paradoxically have a strange way of emphasizing human suffering. Contained in this manner, it sometimes assumes its full tragic dimension. Here is what is said about the lot of copperplate engravers:

They are also exposed to sprains and bruises in the head, arms, legs, and other parts of the body. These are caused by the disposition of the levers which, attached crosswise to the end of the roller, extend more or less far beyond the press and even into the floor space of the workshop. When the press is being turned by a printer who is inattentive or careless, or who has failed to warn his fellow workers who pass too closely to the heated press next to the levers, the workers can be knocked down and very seriously injured.[13]

In the glassworks, the work of the rough polishers had the violence of forced labor. Pajot des Charmes is speaking:[14]

The workers who grind down the mirrors are subject not only to cuts occasioned by the mirrors they are handling every day, but also to apoplexy, for they must rotate their oil stone (a kind of roller weighing 150-186 pounds) over the entire surface of the mirror they have to finish. To do this, they almost always lie flat on their stomach, supported by a bench in order to reach the opposite edge more easily. I have seen some who worked in this manner falling unconscious upon their bench and regaining consciousness only through the help of the strongest stimulants.

Further on, we hear about chalk sifters choking in the dust:

The sifting is usually done in a series of closed rooms and with open sieves; the room is filled with a cloud of chalk-dust that the sifter cannot avoid breathing in. I have seen men and women engaged in this kind of work bring up blood through the nose and the mouth after a few moments. From this one can judge how hard and painful this work is and how greatly it must contribute to shortening the life of this class of mercenaries who are forced to perform it in order to live.

It would be unfair to say that the author is unaware of this tragic aspect. One of the sentences I quoted has all the bitterness of a statement about the human condition: this "painful" work "must" shorten the workers' lives; yet life goes on, while death is being woven, the ineluctable lot of the mercenary who, "in order to live," is forced to submit to it. This vocabulary is taken from two different orders of sentiments, compassion and resignation. A veil of discretion covers the statement as a whole, but it did not deceive the Société Royale de Médecine, which in its report commented on Pajot des Charmes's observations as follows: "Everything seems to conspire against the lives of these unfortunate workers."[15]

What, then, was this "everything" that conspired? It was the workplace, the vapors, and also the motions and the positions involved in working, the manner in which the artisan, in dealing with his materials, was obliged to deform his body, force it, crush it, or simply suffer the impact of injurious materials. The workshop—an objectively death-dealing environment. In the accounts about it written by both the physician and the inspector, one can easily detect the obsessions, sensibilities, and beliefs of the time. *"Air* is what is lacking in most of these workshops." This theme is sounded over and over in the texts, like a harrowing leitmotif. The work areas are too small, the workers toiling side by side have too little breathing space, the windows do not let in enough air, and in winter the workers are afraid of drafts, vapors, and emanations. Physicians and inspectors always suggested the same remedy for this problem, recommending working outside or in large, well-ventilated areas, or else moving the workshop into the open countryside. "Nature" was all the rage; and so everything would be much easier if the manufacturing activities took place outside the city, and if the worker himself were aware of his need for fresh air.

The female wool-pickers [for the task of picking and beating the wool was almost always given to women] are particularly liable to be affected by these indispositions, all the more promptly and severely as they are too thoughtless, or rather too lazy, to open the casement windows, even in summer, so as to establish a strong draft in their workroom which they keep, on the contrary, carefully closed.[16]

The vitalist concept of contemporary medicine, the conviction that the air constantly carries miasmas and impurities capable of making the body ill and propagating disease, runs through all the texts like an obsession. Moreover, it was felt that the people had to be educated to this reality, that they had to be told to circulate the air, to air out their living space: "Laundry must be hung out in the open air. . . . I believe that washerwomen should be relegated to the suburbs of the big cities and no longer be permitted to live in narrow little streets," advises the *Dictionnaire des sciences médicales.*[17] As for quarry workers, they ought to "work with their backs to the wind, so that the dust will be carried away from their faces."

Candlemakers melted their tallow in airless cellars. "They are frequently incommoded by the coal fumes of their furnaces." The solution is simple:

"They would be better off by themselves in the open countryside." Hemp dressers contracted asthma; let them "work outside, with their backs to the wind, and drink soothing marshmallow tea." So, too, for the leather dressers: "Cleanliness and work in open air will remedy the principal impairments that can endanger the leatherworkers' health." Metal gilders would avoid being poisoned by harmful fumes if they were willing to do the scraping in the open air rather than in their workshops.

Moreover, convulsive tremors due to continuous handling of mercury and the inhalation of dangerous mercurial fumes are cured by "living in a place that has pure air." The air purifies everything, protects against any disease, as long as it is good and free of any unhealthy emanation. If the workers cannot breathe in the workshop, let them open the windows, let them work outside. In fact, the artisan may be suffering from a simple lack of hygiene. The tone is undisturbed, the assertions are simple, the answers come automatically, there is no need for complicated reasoning. They need air. All the more so as their bodies, themselves, when they are working, fill the air with harmful exhalations: "In the summer, all the workers of these different workshops give off an unbearable smell, enough to make them sick."[18] Small workshops, annoying fumes, and now body odors, exhalations, effluvia. Triply vitiated in this manner, their air becomes life threatening, so that there is no question that it must be replaced by a healthful air and restored to its essential function, which is to be the breath of life.

Women in particular give off unhealthy odors, especially at the time of their menstrual flow. At that period they contribute to the impurity of the air even more than men. Why, they even cause the color bath in cloth workshops to curdle!

I must not end this article about the manufacture of heavy cloth without mentioning the influence of the bodily emanations of men and women, especially the latter at the time of their indisposition, if it coincides with the preparation of the white and blue bath. . . . If a woman in her critical time were to come even briefly into a room where the bath is set up, it would be enough to make the bath curdle.[19]

Swollen legs, dislocated wrists, trembling hands, nervous spasms, pierced fingers, kidney trouble: the body and its members were used harshly in working, to the point of being deformed and becoming useless. Pajot des Charmes mentions all the infirmities brought about by working; whether benign or irreversible, they constitute a long, monotonous list in which they are virtually impossible to differentiate. It is as if working necessarily brought about injuries, severe or slight.

The rough polishers of mirrors were subject not only to apoplexy "but in addition exposed to the discomforts resulting from the constant dampness of their feet and lower legs, which are wet summer and winter from the water that continuously runs down from the bench on which they work."[20]

In cloth making, the workers who pulled or lifted the wool cloth by chains "suffer considerably from performing this task from morning to night, always standing up. Most of the time, these are children, who will some day replace the weavers whom they serve."[21] In the same trade the wool carders risked having their fingers pierced through. "Even though they are usually very dexterous, they sometimes do pierce their fingers all the way through when handling the comb with its very pointed, sharp, and always long and extremely hot teeth. Although they suffer considerably when this happens, some of them nonetheless, lacking other means of subsistence, continue their work, trying to be more careful in doing it."[22]

But of all the cloth workers, the croppers ran the greatest risk, "being exposed to dislocating or spraining their left wrist as well as to considerable swelling of the muscles under the arm pits. . . . I have several sad examples of this."[23] The warpers or teaselers, by contrast, were exposed only to the "slight inconvenience of receiving cuts or abrasions on their fingers from the constant rubbing of the wool."[24]

The most serious cases were unquestionably those of the gilders, about whom we hear not only from Pagot des Charmes but also from Beerenbrock, physician at Montpellier.[25]

They become subject to generalized trembling of the fingers, hands, and legs, attended by lightheadedness and dizziness; . . . we have seen very young females already affected for this reason, even though they had worked in gilding for only a few years or months. This ailment is not absolutely incurable if the patients can be persuaded to leave their craft in time.

Surely, the most tragic aspect of all this is the fact that one becomes accustomed to these observations and the enumeration of these discomforts.

A Necessary Humanitarianism: The Workers' Health Must Be Preserved

The energy expended by Pajot des Charmes in the detailed description of every last discomfort observed was grounded in more than scientific curiosity. As deputy inspector of workshops, his assignment involved more than that, being of a political nature as well. Workshops had to be efficient but also well ordered; and sickness (or injury) amounted to a kind of disorder. It must be stopped, for it would be scandalous to permit so indispensable a population to founder in misery.

The texts of Pajot des Charmes have one thing in common with those of his contemporaries—physicians or not—who dealt with the same subject: they always approach the subject at different, overlapping levels that are difficult to separate out. Discussing one and the same aspect of a problem, they may imperceptibly shift from humanitarian concern to a rather severe condemnation of an overly careless working class, having earlier evoked the greed of the entrepreneurs. Convictions, a priori judgments, moral considerations, ideology, and personal sensibilities confer upon these texts a character that is coherent only to the extent that it gives perfect expression to the ambiguities and contradictions experienced by the enlightened elites of the time: poverty is necessary, but it must never be permitted to degenerate into wretchedness, since this would bring both dishonor and danger to the nation.

Certain authors considered the poor a fact of life; others even considered them a necessity, an indispensible component of society. They must be given relief but must remain poor; they must not be permitted to sink into wretched helplessness, and they must retain a modicum of dignity. The well-being of humanity demands that this matter be attended to.

The Poor in a State are rather like the shadows in a painting, they make for a necessary contrast that is sometimes bemoaned by humanity, yet is in keeping with the design of Providence. Surely the ambition, vanity, and whimsy of men have brought about the distressing distinctions that are found among them, but it is wisdom to uphold them. It is necessary, then, that the poor exist, but they must not be wretched. The wretched are a shame to humanity, while the poor are part and parcel of political order and economy: it is because of them that abundance reigns in the cities . . . and that the arts are flourishing. Do not the many advantages to be drawn from the poor demand that they be given at least enough to bear their harsh condition with patience?[26]

This significant text opens Dr. Hecquet's book about medical care for the poor. Written as a preface in 1740, it is a perfect exposition of the reasons why mankind cannot permit wretched poverty to take over: it would be shameful to do so; moreover, some relief must be provided if the poor are to tolerate their condition without revolting. Indeed the poor, by their work, permit others to enjoy abundance. The moral order and the political order exist side by side, they mutually support each other, and in a sense refer to each other, lined up in such a way that they sharpen the contours of a schema that no one would challenge. Philanthropy and humanitarian inclinations, moreover, make it possible not to accuse Nature of being unfair: "There are men in society evil-minded enough to accuse Nature, that benevolent mother of all creatures, of having been negligent in her concern for the human race."[27] To accuse Nature or the social order is a vain undertaking; these writers are only interested in providing relief. Pajot des Charmes was in the mainstream of the sensibility of his time when he tried to convince the Société Royale that it would be useful to alleviate the misery of the printers in copperplate engraving. "The man who transfers faithful images of the great masters' paintings onto vellum and paper"[28] fulfills a cultural function, for which society is necessarily indebted to him. It must, therefore, watch over him. This is right and necessary for, among other things, the nation's cultural prestige is at stake. "It is incumbent principally upon medicine to deliver this unfortunate class of workers. . . . There is no doubt that the Société Royale de Médecine would be able to find a great variety of means, one more advantageous than the next, and all most appropriate, for implementing the humanitarian aims of which this illustrious company never loses sight, if it were to decide that this work should become the object of a special program."

Humanitarian thinking, perhaps because of its ideological content, sometimes has the unfortunate characteristic of being totally inadequate—inadequate to the goal it has set for itself, inapplicable to the circumstances, out of line even, and so completely ill-founded as to become harmful because it is out of phase and based on misconceptions and ignorance. Being out of phase is one of the ways of being—consciously or unconsciously—irresponsible and distant. The philanthropist's way.

Dr. Buchan's book on domestic medicine[29] contains some astonishing lines about ill-ventilated workshops and workers riveted to bad postures by their work. "I have already noted that these workers are often sick, the reason being that they are constantly bent over. They must therefore . . . change their posture as often as possible; . . . they ought to leave their work from time to time and go walking, *horseback riding,* and running." Such a statement could be called impudent. Yet there is a certain innocence here, a certain lack of sophistication. In a footnote Buchan adds: "I realize that this advice cannot be given to all workers; . . . a horse would entail expenses beyond their means." No matter, they need exercise and, if they want to reach a serene old age, "they must be convinced that it is of utmost importance for them to combine some recreation with their work, and consequently that they must only work for a few hours at a stretch, then take a walk or run."[30]

Walking and running, "working with their backs to the wind," are so many inapplicable good intentions, so many irresponsible ways of giving advice. "We shall put forth some ideas concerning the means of preserving the health of this useful class of men, and we hope that some of them will be wise enough to pay attention." This is the innocence of authors who are convinced that they are right. They know what it takes to maintain good health, and they tell the world. It is up to the workers to follow their advice—if they are wise.

The physicians' learning is distant, they have a way of saying what is good and what is bad that to some extent shields them from being overly burdened with responsibility for the poor classes. And if, indeed, anyone is responsible, it is usually the workers themselves. The texts of Pajot and others constantly play upon this ambiguous interrelation. The working conditions are harsh, but the workers are overly negligent; impeccable conduct would give them better health, which would enable them to withstand the harshness of the workshop more easily. To place the blame on those who project a highly visible, painful, and indeed almost unbearable image of their condition is to dominate that image, so that it is no longer frightening and can be put to use. This is the path unconsciously taken by the humanitarians; moral notions are often paramount in their vocabulary to the point of permeating the text as a whole. Everything fits together neatly to add the worker's guilt to the causes of diseases and injuries. "Most of the diseases affecting them are usually caused only by their lack of attention, both to the foods they eat and to certain precautions that would protect them from a thousand accidents."[31]

The most unbearable finding, finally, and above all the most dangerous, is to realize how dirty the artisans are. Dirt breeds disease: if the poor kept cleaner, they would avoid many a disease.

Generally speaking, all the workers who habitually work with and handle the greasy wool to be used in the making of heavy cloth have pale, livid, or ashen complexions, a difformity that is compounded by the many colors that always mark their faces; one can imagine how all the different causes of uncleanliness, in their workshops and in their homes, contribute to causing skin diseases, among others those that are known in various places, especially among poor people, under the name of sweating sickness or prickly heat.[32]

It is one thing to become dirty in the pursuit of one's work, another to live in filth, which is flagrantly wrong; there is nothing wrong with being poor, but at least this should not offend other people's sight or sense of smell. "Cleanliness is certainly the workers' least common characteristic."[33] "The charcoal burners should use baths and ablutions, but it must be said that this is the least of their concerns."[34] Uncleanliness is represented in the learned discourse of the period in a twofold manner: it not only results from wretched poverty but also from misconduct. "It will not be easy to put a stop to their uncleanliness, because it is a consequence of their wretched poverty and their misconduct."[35]

The artisan's misconduct has many facets, being made up of negligence, slovenliness, and foolish acts that are frowned upon by the wise and condemned by the learned. In the unwholesome atmosphere of the workshops, the worker drinks too much wine instead of refreshing himself with water; after work he hurries to the tavern, which leads him to nothing but bad company and bad acts; at home he will gorge himself on bad greases instead of eating a balanced diet that would bring relief to his stomach, already uncomfortably compressed by the positions taken in working with machinery. Pajot des Charmes speaks at length about these forms of behavior, while in Panckoucke's *Dictionnaire des sciences médicales* the descriptions of artisans always mention the vices that are attributed to them: "Generally speaking, the workers in the baking trade are often sick—they are seen in great numbers in hospitals, and this is due not only to the demanding work of their trade but also to their custom of working during the night. Moreover, the bakers are very given to wine-drinking, and their apprentices often lead a dissolute life.[36]

The artisan is poor, which is why he is dirty and irresponsible, which is why he becomes ill. The reasoning is logical, flawless, fascinating almost in its direct, unwavering approach, leading step by step to a reassignment of responsibilities. The artisans are to be blamed, to some extent, for becoming ill in the first place. What is more, once they are ill, they refuse to take care of themselves until they are well, out of an excessive greed for money. Thus, the gilders attacked by convulsive trembling upon contact with mercury fumes should know enough to quit their craft earlier than they do. "This ailment is not absolutely incurable if the patients can make up their minds to quit their craft early; but this is rare, for poverty and greed commonly make them come back to it as soon as they feel better; and the more often they backslide, the more the remedies lose their effectiveness."[37]

This succession of disorders that leads to illness and aggravates the misery of a useful population has one rather serious effect that greatly concerns our authors. Ramazzini was the first to speak of it: "The unfortunate artisans, finding dire diseases where they had hoped to draw their own and their families' livelihood, die detesting their thankless occupation."[38] The degradation of the world of crafts must not go this far: it must not lead the worker to detest his occupation; he must not consider it thankless and thereby see nature as hostile to him. When it comes to this, the order of things is upset, and danger threatens. To hate one's work is to become fierce and dangerous. To hate one's work is to open a most disturbing rift in the natural underpinnings of a system founded on the duality of the well-to-do class versus the poor and useful class. A poverty that is necessary to the established order must tolerate its condition without detesting anyone.

At this precise point in the reasoning, the responsibility of the dominating members of society again comes to the fore: the way is long but clear. Having marked the distance between the upper classes and the artisans and proven, once and for all, a certain guilt on the part of the worker, the man of learning reasserts his responsibility and his power. The fault is not all his, for he knows that the worker himself compounds his misfortune; which is why he must be taught to live differently, but also be protected by the necessary safety measures. The assumption that the artisan bears the guilt for his suffering justifies a new kind of domination, bearing the stamp of morality and "charity." Physicians, inspectors of workshops, and their likes are faced with a world to be educated and protected; it is at this level that they exercise their responsibility and their humanitarianism. It is at this level that they respond with a sensibility that by no means impairs their power. It is a sensibility, moreover, that permits them to judge the heads of certain enterprises rather severely. Many improvements can be made immediately by directors of establishments if they will only take the trouble, even if it entails changing the well-entrenched routine of their procedures. "Consider that with the safety precautions indicated [above], which are not too costly in relation to their importance, it would have been possible on many occasions to preserve the valuable days of the head of a family, thereby delivering from indigence and wretchedness a mother and her weeping children."[39]

To prevent danger, to expose the workers to fewer hazards, is not only to be humane but to be efficient. "It is very much in their interest to preserve their workers' health," wrote the editors reporting on Pajot's memoranda. Everything possible must be done to preserve this necessary world of the artisans. For example, the artisans employed in mirrorworks and glassworks are particularly vulnerable to apoplexy and hemorrhages. Glass making involves the use of chalk, which must be sifted. The "sifter" works in such a thick cloud of chalk dust that he chokes and sometimes spits blood. "One could easily avoid any kind of danger by making sure that these ingredients are sifted out of doors. . . . The expense involved would be quite moderate, and moreover would contribute greatly to the preservation of persons who can be of service to their establishments."[40] If it turns out that no immediate improvement in the workshop can be envisaged, it should at least have facilities for administering first aid to the injured; they should be treated even if they are not protected. Here, once again, is Pajot des Charmes, writing about glassworkers:

One can therefore never sufficiently exhort the entrepreneurs of the larger establishments located in towns or in the forests of the countryside to have on the premises, if not a medical practitioner, then at least a stock of instruments or drugs that are needed for administering first aid—which is always the most important—to workers who are drowning or suffocating and to those who are suffering the ill effects of their work or their imprudence.[41]

The discourse here is of an ambiguous clarity; its statements form a coherent pattern even when they contradict each other. Respect for the "system" is paramount: do not change the order of things, but have on hand what you need to repair the inevitable damages produced by both the working conditions and imprudent behavior. The hospital next to the factory. Water by the fire.

Exhorting the entrepreneurs is also to spur them on to become involved in their workers' education. The safety of working bodies necessarily begins with asserting authority over these same bodies. Poor people, ignorant by nature, do not know what they must do to survive. They must be taught. To teach is to lay down rules, to tie the learner to a discipline, and then to make sure that this discipline is followed. To make men's bodies "docile"[42] is also to protect them from illness, although the need for charity remains unchanged. The language in which Dr. Hecquet speaks about the poor is revealing: "It is true that *docility* on their part would be necessary; but in addition, those who are in charge of charitable organizations would have to make some efforts for bringing useful relief to families when the need for it arises; but to what lengths in the service of the poor will one not go when spurred on by the charity of Jesus Christ."

A first concern is to do away with dirt. Educating men's bodies to cleanliness is accomplished by watching for irregular behavior of any kind, imposing and enforcing strict rules, and punishing any disregard of these rules. Cocqereau, who reported to the Société Royale on one of Pajot des Charmes's memoranda, approved of this slow work of subjecting men's bodies, a task that had to be accomplished if order and health were to reign in the workshops.

Here again, we must address ourselves to those who guide them and pay them. It is incumbent upon the entrepreneur of the workshop to supervise the premises; it is also incumbent upon him to *demand* that his workers have reasonably clean linen and work clothes, and to give orders for withholding enough of their daily wages to take care of their clothes and replace them. The workers will submit to these regulations once they realize that they can enter a workshop and work there only under these conditions.[43]

Once the workshop has become a supervised space, it will also become an efficient space: the cleanliness demanded of him will save the poor, and therefore submissive, worker from disease. His health and his submissiveness will result in public tranquillity. More difficult to control are his eating habits, for he eats outside the mill. In this area, a great deal of advice and admonition must be given.

I am convinced that if the poor could be made to return to the use of vegetables, there would be less illness among them; and that those who do become ill would regain their health more rapidly, so that less time would elapse before they are well enough to attend to their occupation and to the raising of their children.[44]

Firmness is all the more necessary here, as the poor too often do not want to listen to advice intended to serve their well-being. Strenuous efforts are therefore needed to combat their reticence; a way must be found to impose a balance that is totally lacking in the lives of the poor. And here again, the learned discourse unconsciously sidesteps the contradictions inherent in its approach: the poor are not disposed toward a balanced life, so that it must be balanced for them; their useful poverty must be preserved yet also alleviated. The reasoning pursues its course, avoiding all pitfalls, and proceeding without offending charitable notions of welfare or jeopardizing the principles of productivity and public order.

Persons engaged in charitable endeavors must give free rein to their zeal, and at the same time they must arm themselves with patience and firmness in order to overcome . . . the ill-humor of those who, in their overwhelming state of dejection, (a normal result of poverty and illness), are often loath to take to heart what is suggested to them for their own good.[45]

In the final analysis, any discourse on the body and on disease is a discourse on behavior and on order. The texts we have examined here are no exception. Nor are they meant to be. Every line, every word, every reasoning pursued encompasses very diverse levels of thinking. One and the same sentence strikes several different chords, yet all of them have only one aim: to make the city peaceful, to make working bearable. The varied discourse of the eighteenth century already foreshadowed what was later to be found in nine-teenth-century books, such as Durand's *La Condition des ouvriers de Paris de 1789 à 1841:*

The way of life of the worker remains simple in the countryside. If he suffers, he resigns himself to God's will, because he has religion . . . ; the worker who, in Paris, covets *something else* beyond the work that brings his daily bread and assures him and his family of food, clothing, and a healthful and convenient dwelling, *becomes dangerous to public tranquillity.*[46]

A public tranquillity was already being fashioned out of a certain docility of working bodies and a specific discipline. This was the beginning of a long-term development.

NOTES

1. Bartolomeo Ramazzini, *Essai sur les maladies des artisans* (Paris, 1777). Translated from the Latin by Fourcroy. It is a book of 577 pages, with an introduction by the translator.

2. Philippe Hecquet, *La Médecine, la chirurgie et la pharmacie des pauvres,* ed. Lacherie, 3 vols. (Paris, 1740).

3. Dr. G. Buchan, *Médecine domestique, ou traité complet des moyens de se conserver en santé, de guérir et prévenir les maladies, par le régime et les remèdes simples,* trans. Duplanil, 5 vols. (Paris, 1775).

4. See the list in the French edition of Ramazzini.

5. Preserved in 200 boxes in the library of the Académie de Médecine, rue Bonaparte, Paris.

6. *Société Royale de Medecine* (hereafter SRM) 122, no. 30

7. SRM 140

8. SRM 174: *Mémoire sur les dangers auxquels sont exposés les teinturiers de grand et de petit teint; Mémoire sur les maladies et incommodités des ouvriers employés dans les manufactures de grande et de petite draperie; Mémoire sur les maladies et incommodités auxquelles sont exposés les ouvriers de verrerie et particulièrement ceux de glacerie* (1787, preserved together with a subsequent report by the Société); *Mémoire sur les maladies et incommodités auxquelles sont exposés les imprimeurs en taille douce* (read on 4 April 1788 to the Société, which published a long report about it).

9. Idem, *Mémore . . . draperie,* p. 13

10. SRM, Report on Pajot des Charmes's *Mémoire . . . verrerie,* SRM 174.

11. Recall that S. A. Tissot could take an interest in writing about the health of literary men and members of high society (1768-70).

12. Ramazzini, *Essai,* author's preface.

13. Pajot des Charmes, *Mémoire . . . imprimeurs,* SRM 174.

14. Idem, *Mémoire . . . verrerie.*

15. SRM, Report on Pajot des Charmes, *Mémoire . . . verrerie,* SRM 174.

16. Pajot des Charmes, *Mémoire . . . draperie,* SRM 174, p. 2.

17. *Dictionnaire des sciences médicales* (Paris: Panckoucke, 1818), vol. 30, s.v. "Maladies des artisans."

18. Pajot des Charmes, *Mémoire . . . draperie,* SRM 174, p. 5.

19. Ibid., p. 7

20. Idem, *Mémoire . . . glacerie,* SRM 174, p. 13

21. Ibid., p. 12.

22. Ibid., p. 9.

23. Ibid., p. 6.

24. Ibid., p. 6.

25. SRM 140, *Maladies des doreurs* (1780), by Beerenbrock, physician at Montpellier.

26. Hecquet, *La Médecine des pauvres.*

27. Ramazzini, *Essai,* author's preface.

28. Pajot des Charmes, *Mémoire . . . imprimeurs,* SRM 174.

29. Buchan, *Médecine domestique.*

30. Buchan, *Médecine domestique,* 1: 122, 134.

31. Cf. Hecquet, *La Médecine des pauvres,* vol. 2.

32. Pajot des Charmes, *Mémoire . . . draperie,* SRM 174, p. 5.

33. *Dictionnaire des sciences médicales,* vol. 40.

34. Ibid.

35. SRM, Reports on Pajot des Charmes's mémoires, SRM 174.

36. *Dictionnaire des sciences médicales,* vol. 30, s.v. "Boulangers."

37. SRM 140, *Maladies des doreurs.*
38. Ramazzini, *Essai,* author's preface.
39. Cf. Pajot des Charmes, *Mémoire . . . glacerie,* SRM 174, p. 20.
40. Ibid., p. 6.
41. Ibid., p. 20.
42. M. Foucault, *Surveiller et punir* (Paris, 1975), p. 137 (English translation by A. M. Sheridan Smith, *Discipline and Punish* [New York, 1977]).
43. Coquereau, *Rapport sur le mémoire de Pajot des Charmes concernant les maladies des imprimeurs en taille douce, 22 juillet 1788.*
44. Hecquet, *La Médecine des pauvres,* vol. 2.
45. Ibid.
46. Durand, *De la condition des ouvriers de Paris de 1789 à 1841* (Paris: Gros, 1841), pp. 189-90.

6

The Structure of the Hospital System in France in the Ancien Régime

Muriel Joerger

In the second half of the eighteenth century a generous share of the criticism leveled against the established institutions concerned the hospitals. Yet the attacks directed against them were all the more intense and contradictory, indeed all the more passionate, as these institutions were not well known. About their internal organization, about that "identity" in which each of them was "clothed,"[1] only bits and pieces wrenched from administrations jealous of their power trickled through to the outside. More curiously, especially since a large part of the critics objected implicitly or quite openly to their excessive numbers—France being the country where hospitals were said to have "multiplied the most"[2]—"their absolute and positive number is unknown."[3] After twelve surveys conducted in the course of the eighteenth century,[4] Necker himself, despite his personal interest in this matter, arrived at an astonishing approximation, claiming that on the eve of the Revolution France had "more than 700 hospitals and about 100 establishments of three or four beds founded by private persons."[5]

When, beginning in 1789, the general reform movement gathered momentum, the much-discussed problem of hospitals was placed on the agenda as a matter of course. A file concerning their number—an indispensable first step toward any projected reform—was opened in 1790 and closed before it was completed in 1792. Nonetheless, it constitutes the first quantitative approach to a problem that hitherto had often been treated in the abstract. This is the file I should like to use in my attempt to grasp the major features of the structure of the hospital system in France at the end of the Ancien Régime.

Annales, E.S.C. 32 (September-October 1977): 1025-51. Translated by Elborg Forster.

To be sure, the question of hospitals, which at the time received old people, abandoned children, beggars, or the sick, has been treated repeatedly in the last few years in studies that have gradually shed more light on the Ancien Régime's relationship with its poor.[6] It is also central to studies describing the changeover from a medicine based on words to a scientific medicine elaborated at the patient's bedside[7] or to the detailed analysis of the functioning of a particular establishment.[8] But the question has never been considered as a "national" development.

In view of the sources at my disposal I should indicate at the outset that my findings are rather modest: what I am offering here is a rough statistical approach, a somewhat dubious geographical overview of the system of hospitals in Ancien-Régime France, an overview, further, that is not easy to keep in focus. Nevertheless, it is worth looking at, even if it is not totally clear, because its very complexity bespeaks its many implications, which are of great interest in themselves. And while it is indeed true that, to quote Jacques Tenon's well-known dictum, "hospitals are the measure of a civilization,"[9] they also reflect the image of a society, which thus becomes a little better known whenever its hospitals are studied.

Sources, Problems, Methods

In December 1791, the Committee on Public Relief (*secours public*) of the Legislative Assembly[10] launched a national survey designed to "acquaint it with the situation of hôtels-Dieu, hospitals, hospices, and other charitable establishments" existing in each municipality.[11] The information that could be derived from this survey has almost totally disappeared from the official records, but it happens to be included in the personal papers of Jacques Tenon, the first person to serve as chairman of this committee.[12] While this source constitutes the first serious approximation of the number of hospitals in France that could be obtained at that time, its use gives rise to a number of problems that I shall summarily evoke here, together with the decisions I have made.

In the first place, the lists of hospitals in the Tenon papers (*Fonds Tenon*) are not reliable, since they were compiled from departmental lists based on frequently scattered and outdated information gathered by the committee on mendicity of the preceding Assembly.[13] Intended to be carefully studied and brought up to date by the local authorities, the lists do not furnish the detailed figures for the totality of establishments that would provide a reliable indication —at least for houses that took in patients—of guaranteed provincial facilities. As they stand, these lists give the number of beds as requested by Paris, and not those actually counted.[14] Before I could use these lists, which were known, even by their authors, to be incomplete and full of errors pending their verification,[15] I systematically checked the information they provided against information from other sources[16] limited to the period 1750-92.

The problem involving the statistical data is compounded by the complex nature of an institution that, designated by a wide variety of words[17] that rarely coincided with a specific meaning, undertook—generally under one roof—very diverse charitable tasks. In a Christian civilization, the hospital, being an outstanding testimony to its founder's faith, took charge of saving bodies as well as souls;[18] and by the same token was invested with as many functions as there are ills and perils threatening mankind. Imprisoned, as it were, by the considerable extension of the word *hospital,* Tenon had concerned himself with a very large group of "charitable establishments," including, for example, "houses providing help in the home" or "combating the fragility of youth." Faced with this imprecisely outlined mass, I decided to limit my study to *civilian hospitals with beds.*[19] These now had to be divided into three categories —hospitals, hôtels-Dieu, and "general hospitals"—on the basis of the three main functions that the hopitals, whatever their actual work and their name, seemed to fulfill in the eighteenth century: providing help, caring for the sick, and "confining."

The largest category[20] corresponds to the mass of establishments that usually had no particular specialty. Under extremely varied names (though often called "hospitals," so that this name, in quotation marks, will hereafter be used to designate this type of establishment), they provided the entire gamut of welfare services for the parish where they were located, and often for that parish only. Taking in invalids, incurables, old people, abandoned children, and the sick, they also organized help in the home, the distribution of food and clothing, and even the teaching of poor children.

By contrast, the hôtels-Dieu, to use the name that most often designated this type of hospital, were normally reserved for the sick, even if they sometimes had to assume financial or administrative responsibility for other charitable services. Generally open to all, without regard to geographical origin, they did exclude the incurables,[21] and, depending on the establishment, patients suffering from venereal disease or scrofula, the mad, and pregnant girls or women.

Completing this triptych of hospitals of the Ancien Régime, the general hospitals, founded in the seventeenth century to "confine" beggars, had by the eve of the Revolution assumed the appearance of immense "hospices"[22] whose basic inmates were virtually indistinguishable from those who, generally speaking, populated the "hospitals." Moreover, they took in those categories of patients that were rejected by the hôtels-Dieu. In fact, they constituted, especially in the eighteenth century, something approaching central regulatory agencies for a society where the abandonment of children had become more and more prevalent and where the economic circumstances of the time, related to a long-unrecognized demographic expansion, had led to widespread and quasi-institutionalized unemployment. Also to be found in the general hospitals were abandoned children who, once they reached the age of seven, were no longer cared for by the hôtels-Dieu and individuals cast into poverty by a temporary crisis or an illness.[23] But for all that, they continued to function as the prison wardens of a social order that banished from its stage those who did not bend to its norms; the insane and all those who lived beyond the limits of the sexual ethic were confined there.[24]

Finally, I have sidestepped one last problem connected with my source by casting my study in the departmental framework of the Revolutionary survey. This makes it easier to keep control of the data and also permits me to make use of subsequent information, especially the census of 1806.[25]

This piecemeal approach and the specific choices made—to which I will return later—have enabled me to present a preliminary tally. The highest total of the Tenon papers furnishes a list of 2,326 hospitals, of which 1,833 establishments remain, once military hospitals and hospitals without beds are subtracted. Of these 1,833 hospitals, only 30 percent were listed with their number of beds, which, as I explained above, is the only proof that they actually existed in 1791-92. By adding or subtracting certain establishments on the basis of supplementary sources, I arrived at a figure of 1,961 hospitals. Most importantly, I am able to prove the actual existence of 72 percent of them and to give the number of beds for 61 percent. An improbable source has thus been made to yield historically acceptable data, always provided that their limitations be kept in mind.

To begin with, the number of hospitals remains strictly approximate at the departmental level. In only 55 of the departments was it possible to verify at least 70 percent of the establishments (and this is the minimum figure for obtaining a sufficiently reliable image of reality). For the 27 other departments, this percentage varies between 69 and 50 percent in 18 cases and is even lower for the rest (see map 6.1). This margin of uncertainty is all the more disturbing as a ranking of the departments by decreasing number of hospitals shows that the departments where the fewest establishments can be verified actually had the greatest number. Applied to the two sets of departments where the level of verification was higher or lower than 70 percent, a test[26] designed to determine whether the elements composing the two groups proceed from the same set fortunately yields reassuring results. It appears that, provided the departments of Basses-Alpes, Bouches-du-Rhône, and Var (in other words, Provence), as well as Seine-et-Oise and Seine-et-Marne, are not counted among the total of insufficiently verified departments (less than 70 percent), the latter are as usable for my study as the others; even though, in practice, we should no doubt imagine them as less well endowed than the figures would indicate.[27] As for those that are "not counted," the profusion of hospitals there unquestionably corresponds to a different model, but it is one whose existence is quite certain. In 1847 when the first reliable census of hopitals was taken, these departments were still ahead of all the others;[28] moreover, the great number of hospitals, at least in Provence, is well known by the historians of that province.[29]

The inadequacy of my data has even more serious consequences for the analysis of the number of beds. Recall that only 61 percent of the hospitals indicated their capacity. Furthermore, only forty-three of the departments gave the number of beds for at least 70 percent of their establishments (this being the percentage below which I decided not to count a department at all). Finally, the number of beds is consistently underevaluated. This is true for hospitals and above all for hôtels-Dieu, which constantly and officially "doubled" and even "tripled" their beds; it is also true for the general hospitals, which admitted inmates according to available resources or the severity of a crisis rather than according to the number of beds. In any case, that number was rarely "fixed" and, if it was, always outstripped by demand.[30]

This critical evaluation of my source material does not mean that the statistical tallies, the maps, and the conclusions I shall draw from them should be rejected. Rather, my conclusions should be taken for what, in a modest way, they purport to be: indicators of a general tendency.

The Network of Hospitals: Numbers

ESTABLISHMENTS AND FORM OF RELIEF

The network of hospitals in Ancien-Régime France should first of all be approached in terms of a tally. There were 1,961 hospitals and, for the 61 percent of establishments that indicated their capacity, 86,252 beds. In my opinion, there is no need to challenge these figures in any fundamental sense.

A systematic and painstaking comparison with the plentiful data from an 1847 survey of hospitals[31] leads me to believe that this total of 1,961 hospitals does not exceed the actual number by more than 100-150 units.[32] Given a population of 26 million, this high tally makes for a hospital/population ratio that was never to be reached again. From 0.75 per thousand on the eve of the Revolution it dropped to 0.36 in 1847 and has risen to a figure of 0.69 today.[33] But behind these clear-cut figures there is a network of hospitals totally lacking in geographic and structural unity.

To begin with, the uneven distribution of these 1,961 hospitals created pronounced regional contrasts, with the dividing line running roughly from Saint-Malo to Geneva! Yet it should be added that this trite schema—in which the North does not, however, form a monolith—is strangely broken or modified by the presence of a zone of very heavy concentration of hospitals in the Mediterranean South (in the wider sense) and along a kind of umbilical cord linking the North with the South more or less closely following the river valleys of the Saône and the Rhône. (See map 6.2.)

The general unevenness in the distribution of hospitals is overlaid by an uneven distribution of the different types of establishments. The "hospitals" conform to the geography I have just outlined for hospital establishments as a whole (see map 6.3). General hospitals, though present everywhere (see map 6.4) show a certain predilection for western and central France, while hôtels-Dieu are clustered in the country's northern half (see map 6.5).

Finally, the local geographical distribution of hospitals adds another element of diversity to the two I have already identified. The nature of the hospital was

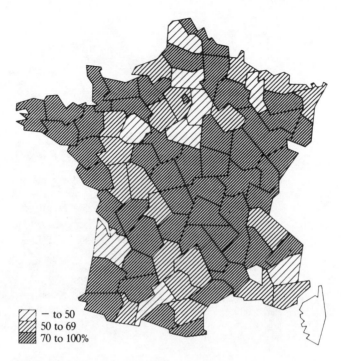

− to 50
50 to 69
70 to 100%

Map 6.1. Level of Verification of Data

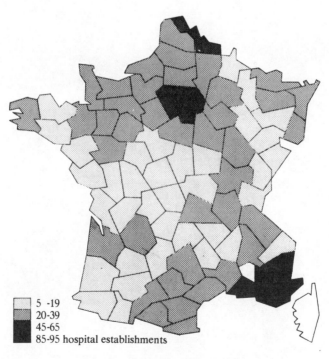

5 -19
20-39
45-65
85-95 hospital establishments

Map 6.2. Distribution of All Hospital Establishments by Department

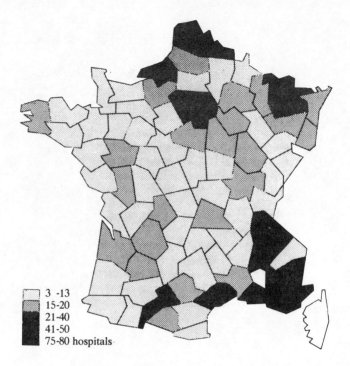

3 -13
15-20
21-40
41-50
75-80 hospitals

Map 6.3. Distribution of "Hospitals" by Department

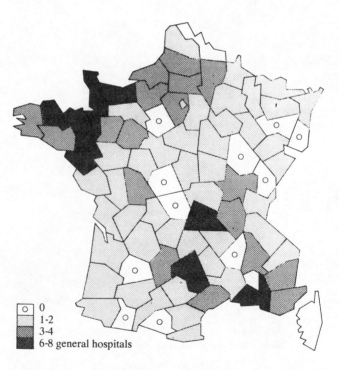

○ 0
1-2
3-4
6-8 general hospitals

Map 6.4. Distribution of General Hospitals by Department

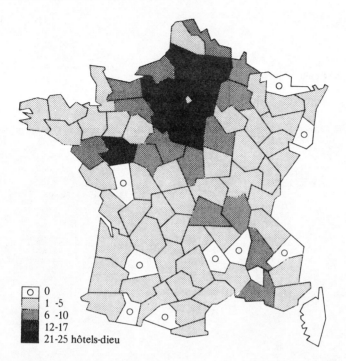

Map 6.5. Distribution of Hôtels-Dieu by Department

essentially a function of the agglomeration in which it was located. The vast mass of small agglomerations claimed most of the "hospitals," for it turns out that 52.71 percent of the localities that had at least one hospital had less than 2,000 inhabitants and that 11.39 percent had less than 1,000 inhabitants. The hôtel-Dieu already appears as an almost exclusively urban institution, since only 33.85 percent of the localities counting a hôtel-Dieu had less than 2,000 inhabitants. The general hospitals, intended from the outset as "regional" institutions and also as a means of reducing the pressure of destitute people on the principal cities, were clustered to a large extent (57.62 percent) in urban centers of more than 7,500 inhabitants, although—and this is worth mentioning here already—they did not totally shun more modest localities either. (See fig. 6.1.)

In the same manner as its geographic distribution, the underlying structure of the network of hospitals testifies to a certain imbalance. This structure was essentially constituted by the "hospitals" (1,398 units, or 71.23 percent of the total), while the hôtels-Dieu represented only one-fifth of the total number of establishments (387 units, or 19.78 percent). There is nothing odd about this disproportion, for the hôtels-Dieu, being "specialized" institutions, were not as "practical" as the "hospitals." Moreover, the hôtels-Dieu, however rudimentary they may have been at times, still did imply a fairly complex infrastructure (pharmacy, morgue, and so forth) and a vaguely specialized staff that in some measure—and increasingly so as the eighteenth century progressed—called

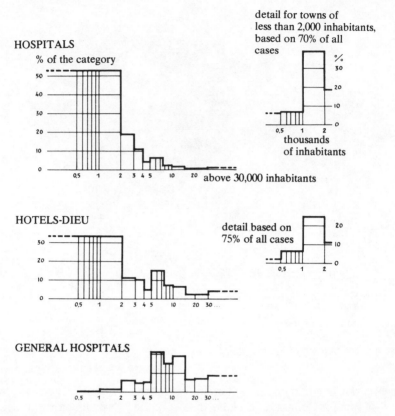

Figure 6.1. Distribution of the Different Types of Hospital According to Size of Agglomeration.

for the presence of physicians who, as recent studies have shown, were urban notables.[34] The general hospitals, finally, were of recent origin, and while they accounted for only 9.02 percent of the network of hospitals as a whole, they nevertheless reached the rather remarkable total of 177 establishments (see fig. 6.2). Taken at their face value, these maps may seem to testify to the weight of traditional charity, of the kind that was practiced by the many "hospitals" that, like those of the Middle Ages, refused to distinguish between moral or material distress and physiological distress. But this may well be the afterglow of a reality that no longer existed. The situation looks very different if one studies the number of beds and their use.

One might tend to think that the total capacity of the establishments of the Ancien Régime (recall that 61 percent of them accounted for 86,252 beds) was rather similar to what it was to be fifty years later (a total of 126,142 beds in 1847).[35] But beyond any statistical similarities or dissimilarities, there was a fundamental difference in goals between the old welfare system and the system that subsequently was to come into being.

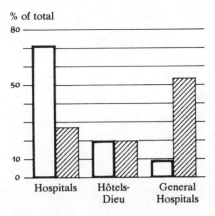

Note: Blank column = number of establishments; shaded column = number of beds

Figure 6.2. Distribution of the Different Categories of Hospital and of Hospital Capacity
for Each Entry

The "hospitals," despite their number, offered only 27.12 percent of the
beds (see fig. 6.3). The reason is that in almost 40 percent of the cases (39.15
percent; see fig. 6.3) they had a capacity of less than ten beds. The "hospitals"
were thus quite often no more than hovels, such as they were described in
surveys throughout the eighteenth century, places where a charitable old
woman was in charge of a few pallets and made house calls. They did not
accomplish very much, but were vigorously defended by popular insurrection
or costly lawsuits whenever their abolition was contemplated.

Very much larger as a rule (44.3 percent had between 21 and 80 beds and
11.3 percent had more than 100), the hôtels-Dieu accounted for 19.78 percent
of the total hospital capacity. By adding to this the two-thirds of the "hospital"
beds that may be assumed to have been used for sick patients,[36] one arrives at
a figure that brings the proportion of "medical beds" to 37.80 percent of the
total. This figure is shockingly small considering that as early as 1847 the
compiler of the survey on welfare expressed indignation at the fact that
hospital beds represented only 54.10 percent of the total, and that this
proportion had reached 68.82 percent by 1973. More serious still is the fact
that this figure goes together with a preposterously low ratio of medical beds
to population: It was 0.51 per thousand (rising to 1.32 per thousand by 1847
and reaching 7.9 per thousand in 1973), although it was estimated early on in
the nineteenth century that in order to meet all needs it should be 8 per
thousand, a figure that "is still used as a basis for discussion in recent studes."[37]
These proportions and these ratios explain the references to hospital beds
permanently occupied,[38] to their "doubling" and "tripling," and to the despair
of hospital administrators who had to discharge convalescents too early,

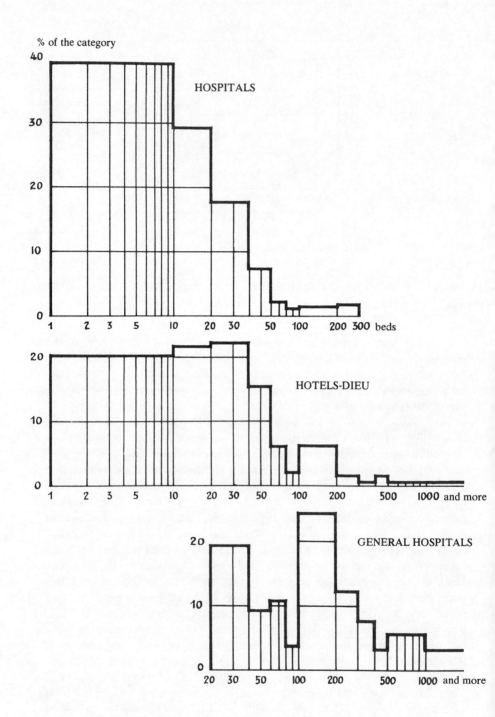

Figure 6.3. Capacity of the Different Types of Hospital

thereby condemning them to relapses. In short, they explain the overcrowding of the hôtels-Dieu despite the terror inspired by the hospital.[39]

The general hospitals, finally, received or "confined," as the case might be, 53.28 percent of the hospitalized population. Most of them, to be sure, were very large (45.96 had between 100 and 499 beds); and some were enormous. Yet the proportion of these establishments having less than 60 beds (28.8 percent) brings to light a kind of general hospital that is as disturbing as the behemoth of the big cities. This was the institution that, for all its provincial mediocrity, propagated and implanted social control in places where one would expect it to be unknown.

Perceived in this manner—that is, through the number of beds—the structure of France's system of hospitals shows its underlying repressive tendency, or rather—since at the end of the eighteenth century real repression was directed only toward certain marginal groups—its regulatory function within the social order. In placing enormous emphasis on relief for the unfortunate (for by adding to the beds of the general hospitals one-third of the beds of the "hospitals" one arrives at a grand total of at least 62 percent of the total hospital capacity earmarked for taking care of the disinherited, which is almost as much as today's hospital beds for the sick), the social system attempted to deal as best it could with the paradoxical problem of a mass of needy people in an expanding country. It was precisely this fundamental feature of the hospital system, one that reflected a social imbalance, that was violently attacked in the second half of the eighteenth century. Some members of the reform-minded elite felt that only hospitals providing medical services were tolerable, and indeed indispensable. But of course welfare establishments, even when conceived in this manner, still perpetuated a system in which there were institutions specifically for the needy—the hospital, which offered "to the poorest patients free of charge the same advantages that are available to richer people"[40]—and other facilities for the well-to-do, where physicians used the hospitals to increase their knowledge.[41] This is why those who favored the hospital, "a wholesale, cut-rate healing machine,"[42] played down its fundamentally conservative aspect by expressing their hope that the gradual disappearance of poverty would eventually do away with the need for it, except for very special medical cases, for foreigners, or for persons without a family.[43]

The structure of France's system of hospitals can thus be understood in a threefold manner. It can be seen in its traditional reality, dominated by the desire to provide indiscriminate charity; in its underlying eighteenth-century reality, marked by its function of upholding the social order; and in its future and already emerging reality as the guardian of the nation's health.

HOSPITALS AND POPULATION

In the eighteenth century the ties that had been established between the French hospital system and the country's demography endowed it with an underlying rationality of which its contemporaries were not aware, for they continued to feel that the hospital was essentially tied to the capricious will of a founder.

At the most encompassing level, the hospitals show the same unequal distribution between North and South as the population:[44] the greatest number of hospitals is found in areas with the highest density of population. Moreover, this correlation also holds, in the North and in the South, on a more modest regional scale that makes it even more striking. French Flanders, Normandy, and, to a lesser degree, Alsace—that is, the great human reservoirs of the well-populated northern part of France—also possessed a maximum number of hospitals. On the other hand, the population densities of central France, the Charente, and Béarn, which were low even when perceived as part of the vast "underpopulated" South, had as a corollary the particularly sparse presence of hospitals. Yet such rough correlations, which do not preclude many local situations that do not fit—and among them Languedoc, Dauphiné, and above all Provence are the most striking—cannot suffice; vague similarities and especially approximate comparisons of absolute figures will not do.

However, statistical calculations systematically centered upon establishing the relation between the number of hospitals at the departmental level and the corresponding population figure have confirmed the general findings outlined above. Provided that the five departments[45] whose behavior was earlier seen to be aberrant are eliminated from the France of 1792, it appears that both the coefficient of correlation and the index of dispersion show an indisputable general relationship between the system of hospitals and demography. (See appendix 1.) Nonetheless, as I indicated earlier, many exceptions did exist. Moreover, it is from those hospital/population ratios that were exceptionally high or exceptionally low in relation to the average ratio (amounting to 0.68 per thousand)[46] that we can learn more about the true lines of strength or weakness of the structure of the hospital system than from the absolute number of hospitals. (See map 6.6.)

Outside of the departments of Haute-Saône (0.33 per thousand) and Rhône-et-Loire (0.34 per thousand) and all of the mountainous areas (Jura, 0.39 per thousand; Cantal, 0.39 per thousand; Basses-Pyrénées, 0.38 per thousand), the zone of France most lacking in hospitals was the West. This zone began in Normandy (even though the absolute number of hospitals there was rather high), continued in Brittany (not counting Finistère), and then ran all along the Atlantic coast. Contrasting with this zone, there were three areas showing very high ratios, as we have already seen on the maps showing the presence of hopitals in general. They were the Paris Basin, the transitional zones toward the western provinces or the Loire, and a very extensive Mediterranean "crescent" of territories that has already been mentioned, although it must henceforth be understood to include the department of Pyrénées-Orientales, where the number of hospitals was small but where the hospital/population ratio has been found to be high.

A systematic investigation of the relation between the number of a department's inhabitants and the number of hospital beds (and it should be kept in

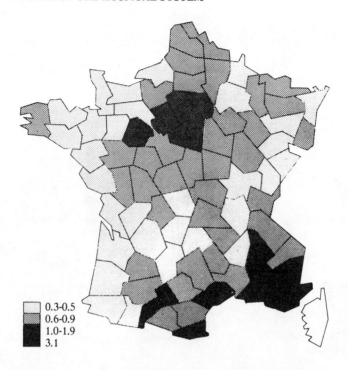

0.3-0.5
0.6-0.9
1.0-1.9
3.1

Map 6.6. Number of Hospital Establishments per 1,000 Inhabitants, by Department

mind that these figures are available for only forty-two departments)[47] also shows a definite connection with the demographic situation, for, as in the case of hospitals, one finds a high index of correlation. Nonetheless, this correlation is less pronounced than for the hospitals themselves, since the calculations show, for example, that the average weighted spread is considerable. (See appendix 1.)

Very incomplete though they are, these data concerning hospital capacity nonetheless enable us to refine the information provided by the hospital/population ratio (see map 6.7). They bring to light pockets of real poverty with respect to hospitals (few hospitals *and* few beds, as in the present departments of Haute-Marne and Côtes-du-Nord and along the entire rim of the Massif Central); on the other hand, they also enable us to discover two areas that compensated for their dearth of establishments with beds/population ratios slightly higher than the average. This was the case in parts of western and central France, that is, two regions of France where the density of general hospitals was by far the highest. In view of this, one may well wonder whether this way of "catching up" represented a massive response to the misery of cold regions or the expression of a repressive mentality that was particularly strong in such isolated areas, and perhaps exacerbated by pervasive poverty.

Above all, the ratio of beds/1,000 people makes it possible to measure the

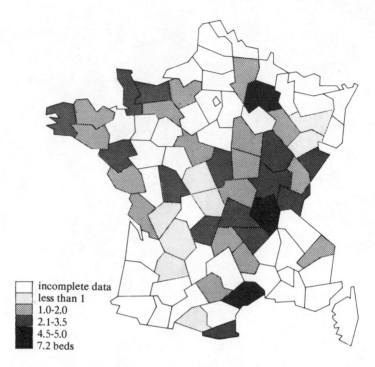

incomplete data
less than 1
1.0-2.0
2.1-3.5
4.5-5.0
7.2 beds

Map 6.7. Number of Beds per 1,000 Inhabitants, by Department

importance of the hospital phenomenon in large cities and the weight of the major population centers in the departmental statistics. For it turns out that the four departments showing the highest ratio of beds/1,000 people owed this privileged position to the presence of large population centers. The absence of Montpellier would have deflated the ratio in the department of Hérault, the difference being between 4.58 and 1.5; without Reims, the ratio in the department of Marne would have been 2.77 rather than 4.84; Caen raised the ratio of Calvados from 1.06 to 3.47; and Lyons raised those of Rhône and Loire from 1.06 to an astonishing 7.24. This list could be lengthened by many departments where a respectable ratio conceals a veritable desert. The existence of the latter is all the more striking as it is in stark contrast with the massive availability in large cities (frequently showing similar ratios: Lyons, 25.05; Reims, 21.49; Montpellier, 28.43; Besançon, 20.48),[48] for the presence of a floating population, though clearly swelling the demand, still does not justify this pronounced imbalance.

The "preparedness" in the area of hospitals (*"armement hospitalier"*),[49] while not rigidly fixed, is clearly related to numerical demographic data and was, moreover, also determined by the distribution of the population. Leaving aside the problem of clustered settlements versus dispersed settlements,[50] I shall deal here only with the coincidence between hospital structures and urban structures. Considering only the presence of hospitals, the correlation between hospital and town matches the ratio of beds/population. Speaking of the various types of hospitals, I have already touched upon the matter of preferential installations in the different types of agglomeration. Adopting the summary statistical definition by which a town is any settlement above 2,000 inhabitants, one might say—speaking now of the total number of hospitals—that 57.27 percent of them were located in towns. And yet, at the end of the eighteenth and the beginning of the nineteenth centuries, these towns contained only 18.8 percent of the French population. Finally, one finds a very marked coincidence between areas of the most pronounced hospital density and areas with the highest number of towns.[51] This phenomenon can be observed along the shores of the Mediterranean, and most clearly in Provence, as well as in French Flanders, in the regions around Paris, and in Champagne in the areas that were to become the departments of Marne, Alsace, and Lorraine.

These statistics and maps only echo the criticism voiced over and over throughout the eighteenth century, and by people from all walks of life,[52] that the rural population was not cared for and that towns were overly privileged when it came to hospitals. This privileged connection between towns and hospitals, while not unknown in the past, is now proven on a national scale. It constitutes a fundamental benchmark for anyone who wants to understand the structure of the hospital system in the Ancien Régime. Henceforth considered a given fact,[53] and in part "natural" for the early-modern period—as it had been in the Middle Ages—this connection was nonetheless also largely determined by historical circumstances.

The connection between towns and hospitals was "natural" because material and physiological distress—which was diluted, as it were, in rural areas—quickly assumed an unbearable and massive character in urban centers, especially since the latter always attracted a part of the down-and-out of the rural world. And in towns the waves of misery could be channeled toward a well-to-do class that was larger or more concentrated there than in the countryside. These were people who in their hearts felt the impact of this spectacle more keenly as they somehow had to come to terms with their own wealth, with the Christian obligation of charity—in short, with God. Urban centers, after all, were the focal points of religious fervor until the end of the eighteenth century.[54] Nonetheless, in specific cases, the visible impact of poverty on a social or economic elite could and did occur outside an urban context, so that the town was not necessarily the only creator of the hospital as an institution. And indeed, until the sixteenth century, many small hospitals had been humbly distributed throughout the countryside.[55]

Only in the sixteenth and seventeenth centuries did a change in sensibility and the assertion of a new political order restrict the phenomenon of hospitals largely to the towns. By the beginning of the seventeenth century, the destruction and the disorders provoked by the Religious Wars and later by the Fronde had thrown the system of hospitals into almost complete disarray.

Paralleling the economic developments of the period, these events also emptied the countryside "in favor" of the towns,[56] leading to an increased concern about the social order that, in conjunction with the weight of new ideas issued from humanistic thinking, was to contribute to taking away from the poor the kind of sacred prestige that had long endowed them with privileged status. As we now know very well, the poor gradually began to appear to the urban elites as carriers of epidemics, possible fomentors of disorder, and potential transgressors against the religious and moral order that the Counterreformation was trying to reconstruct at that time. In this manner, the necessary reorganization of the hospital was precipitated by a rising tide of danger that the authorities would try to avert by a policy of "confinement" in general hospitals. The activities of ambulant missionaries,[57] who stressed the religious component of this new sensibility, led to the foundation of new kinds of establishments that would provide spiritual renewal as well as help for the body. This fundamental development gained so much ground that henceforth no town, no agglomeration exhibiting the characteristics of a town, if only by virtue of the presence within its walls of a certain social elite,[58] could be conceived of without a general hospital or, in its stead, a hospital that was sometimes called by extension "hospital for the Confined."[59] By the beginning of the eighteenth century, only bequests in rural areas were still earmarked for "the poor at liberty;" in the towns bequests usually went to the hospital, which had become the charitable institution *par excellence*.[60]

But the most important consequence of this policy of making the hospital an urban institution was the gradual disappearance from the countryside of the old hospitals. Not only were they deprived of the aid they had often received from the city because donors had come to feel that the urban needs were more pressing, but they also and above all were in conflict with the powers that be. In fact, this urban-directed policy was in keeping with the general approach of a centralizing power wielded by men whose moral and administrative preoccupations were grounded in the same social ethic that informed the attitudes of the social elites scattered throughout the kingdom. The same desire for order was felt at Versailles as in the smallest town. But the national government was determined to guide this desire and consequently to provide the facilities for containing the tide of "idlers" and sufferers in establishments that could be properly registered and supervised. As much in order to carry out this supremely important task as to rationalize its welfare system—and the latter preoccupation was a direct outcome of the former—the central power endeavored to control the enormous charitable *élan* of the Counterreformation by the judicious distribution of letters patent. Above all, it tended to do away with small rural hospitals. Despite popular opposition,[61] these hospitals were often *merged* with urban institutions, and their moneys, on the pretext of poor management, were made to swell the coffers of the new or revived hospitals established everywhere in the kingdom by the state, the municipalites, or the Church. There was no distinction between political order and religious and moral order in this undertaking, in which all parties were involved.

Turgot was the first official figure to speak up, in 1774, against this policy of concentration and to recommend that small hospitals be restored to rural areas totally lacking in facilities.[62] Actually, some medium-sized market towns had already begun to build new hospitals,[63] either because the repressive character of the urban mentality had reached beyond the city dweller or, as so many signs seem to indicate, because the total lack of facilities for the rural population finally made the need for change too evident to be ignored.[64]

The close connection between hospital and town that existed at the end of the eighteenth century emphasizes and illustrates the complexity of the hospital as an institution, for it coincided with the town to the extent that the forces that permanently shaped society originated in an urban milieu. And, for the most part, these forces were indistinguishable from the factors that led to the creation of hospitals. One is indeed justified, therefore, in thinking that the strong and weak points of the hospital system, a mirror image of society, reflected, on a national scale, the regional disparities of France in the Ancien Régime.

Hypotheses

The complexity of an institution that assumed responsibility for peoples' entire lives corresponds to the complexity of the different types of sensibility that seem to me to shed light on certain aspects of the French hospital system.

The hospital's deep concern about the human soul—even at the end of the eighteenth century, though the institution tended to become laicized by then[65] —indicates that religious sensibilities were of prime importance. I might add that the maps showing the distribution of hospitals I was able to draw up are, in my opinion, so clearly related to the efforts at restructuring the network of hospitals made in the early-modern period that it seems legitimate to seek the explanation of this model—partly secular though it was—in the religion of the seventeenth and eighteenth centuries. My starting point is the hypothesis that the geographical pattern and the density of hospitals correspond to what one might call the regional varieties of religious *élan*. Unfortunately, however, the religious sociology of early-modern France, whose inherent complexity is compounded for the time being by the fact that it is still in its infancy, does not, on the national level, provide us with the information that would have constituted our best reference, namely, the quality of religious faith, or at least the indicators that are used to assess it. For that reason, I availed myself of a number of well-known and rather circumscribed criteria, that is, the efforts to combat Protestantism or "paganism," the spread of Jansenism in its early form, and the baroque manifestations of Catholicism. These criteria were to help me identify the regions that experienced exceptional forms of religiosity, which might have temporarily endowed them with a particular *"élan."* For it seemed to me that this *élan*, though not always leading to or reflecting a deeply felt or enduring fervor, was bound to bring men face to face with the demands made by the astonishing Catholic revival of the seventeenth century. Most outstanding among these demands, and more highly valued than ever, was the obligation of good works, particularly charity. This may seem to be a simplistic approach, yet it yields some rather convincing parallels.

The example of the areas where Protestantism had been solidly entrenched, and where the Church embarked very early on a strenuous campaign of reconquest, offers the best illustration of such a connection. For hospitals were much more numerous than they would have been under the logic of a system partly conditioned by population density in Guyenne, Languedoc, Dauphiné, and also Alsace (though the religious and political situation in that province was rather exceptional), all regions where the Reformation had taken an enduring hold. The reason is that the insistence upon charity, of which the hospital was the outstanding expression, was a basic feature of the Catholic reconquest. For it was a matter of anchoring down a religion that stressed as one of its essential tenets salvation through works, precisely one of the points that Protestantism did not accept. Faced with adversaries who, without accepting the obligation of charity as a dogma, had nonetheless developed a special system of mutual help, the Church was challenged to promote a vigorous social program of its own.[66]

This is why ordinary mission territories, where the pressure of the religious authorities was much less constant, geographically more limited, and no doubt less centered on works, did not, like the Protestant areas, show a high and systematic concentration of hospitals. Yet one is tempted to explain the astonishing hospital/population ratios in the Paris region (understood in a very large sense) by the Church's vigorous efforts to strengthen its hold over that area in the eighteenth century. These efforts, described in detail for the diocese of Paris,[67] took the form of sending missionary preachers to every last corner of the area. Many of them were priests of the order of Missions, founded by Saint Vincent de Paul, whose work in the hospital field is well known. Their activities were to bring about the establishment of innumerable "charitable societies" and, I would add on my own since the work I am using as my reference does not deal with this topic, probably also hospitals. Aside from this missionary activity, which was circumscribed in time, it seems obvious to me that the influence of the capital, the seat of many religious orders working within the framework of their diocese or in adjacent areas, was fundamental. Aside from this impact of a militant Catholicism, there is no explanation for the existence in northern France of a zone where the density of hospitals was so great that in the relevant statistical tests it stands out as "atypical."

In certain cases, a rash of hospital foundings seems to testify more to a deep inner impulse than to a response to pressure. The map of the total number of hospital establishments shows, running along the valleys of the Rhône and Saône, a continuous route of densely clustered establishments that subsequently extends into Burgundy and the region of Orleans. Sometimes these densities only serve to produce favorable averages in the hospital/1,000 people ratio of the departments concerned (Saône-et-Loire, 0.82; Côte-d'Or, 0.64), but they do raise the ratios of Yonne (0.82) and especially Loiret (1.22). The massive presence of hospitals may well be related to the facilities offered by nature, for these hospitals were located essentially in a series of valleys surrounded by more or less mountainous and inhospitable areas. Yet this distribution also permits a different hypothesis. For here we find, coinciding rather closely with these areas—especially after 1725—some of the areas that had been touched by Jansenism, which may have been the determining factor.[68] Whatever its ultimate deviances and, in certain cases, its ties with an eventual "dechristianization," Jansenism, with all the religious fervor it implied, was certainly capable of arousing the impulses necessary, in my opinion, to bring about the founding of hospitals on a large scale. The very high concentration of hospitals found in Lorraine, where the existence of an uncompromising variety of Jansenism is an incontrovertible fact[69] (complemented in the department of Meurthe by the high ratio of 0.84), might serve to strengthen this hypothesis.

The new religious—and sociocultural—attitude toward the poor was so fundamental in the matter of hospitals that it left its mark on a national scale. Spreading beyond the elites where it had originated, its success was responsible for nothing less than a new map, that of the general hospitals, and for the basic character of that map, which shows no notable discontinuities in a network that had been so recently established. It is true that, despite their religious roots, the general hospitals were also, as we have seen, the real and symbolic expression of order and rationality, two key notions that the elites used more or less consciously in governing a kingdom in which there was no longer any room for marginal people. The extraordinary practical, if not ideological, success of the general hospital is thus not surprising, any more than the wide distribution of these establishments, which had also brought about a considerable simplification in the old network of "hospitals." And yet new religious sensibilities, important as they were, cannot fully explain the peculiarities of a very complex and multifaceted structure, which must be related to other orders of mentality as well.

There is, for example, a striking connection between the positively Italian or Hispanic[70] profusion of hospitals in Provence, Languedoc, Rousillon, and even French Flanders[71] and the area of France where a baroque sensibility had developed. Surely these were regions where the Catholicism of a remarkable Counterreformation found its most striking, most spectacular, and in extreme cases most exotic expression. Yet here the exemplary nature of the relationship between religious fervor and emphasis on hospital building seems to me less convincing than the existence of a common denominator underlying both these phenomena. The brilliant manifestations of Catholicism in these regions—and we know this at least for Provence and Languedoc, which were to experience a rapid dechristianization in the nineteenth century—were not so much the end result of a deeply felt religion as the expression of the baroque temperament. After all, the taste for the highly visible gesture,[72] which is one of the characteristics of that temperament, was an extremely powerful motive when it came to showing generosity toward a foundation known by everyone. Less palpable, but possibly very important as well, seems to be the impact of another fundamental component of the baroque civilization, namely, its receptivity toward images of physical decrepitude and death. Nowhere were these images more present than in the day-to-day life of hospitals, which may well have attracted their benefactors through the troubled and unconscious working of their sensibilities.

It may be possible to go even further and to think that the rash of hospital foundings in the Provençal South or in Languedoc was also a manifestation of the "imponderable realities"[73] of the temperament of these regions. The need to communicate is certainly one of the essential characteristics of the French Southerner, and this *sociability* found its expression in the almost compulsive desire and the pleasure felt in being together, in founding more or less organized groups where the notion of mutual help could flourish. In the religious context of a Counterreformation that was experienced with great intensity, this notion of mutual help became the *raison d'être* of brotherhoods[74] constituted for the purpose of founding or directing hospitals—which became more numerous for that very reason.

Yet we must not forget that the hospital, beyond its religious, sociological, and even political significance, represented a concrete material effort continually sustained by legacies, gifts, and alms. Although dependent on individual generosity, these donations nonetheless reflected the local possibilities of the donors, and hence a specific moment in the economic development of the region. Moreover, the success of that development also shaped relations within the community and the extent to which individuals were able to respond to the new ideologies that are so important to the subject under discussion here. In the populous north of France (understood in the larger sense), a great many hospitals were established in the area where the "peoples' faculties"[75] [i.e., their economic strength] were already flourishing in the early-modern period. Conversely, certain zones where very low hospital/population ratios testify to a real dearth of hospitals were also those in which the investigators working for the survey of Orry (Controller General in 1745) described poverty and even total indigence. These were regions like the Ardennes, the rim of the Massif Central, or the Vendée. But in fact it would be even easier to cite many examples of a lack of correlation between the cartographic representation of prosperity or poverty and that of hospital/population ratios by department. Southern France, to which one must refer again and again, shows a discrepancy between its relatively modest resources and the number of its hospital establishments, while Normandy shows a discrepancy between its widespread prosperity and practices amounting to abandoning people to their fate. There is no question that the day-to-day management of a hospital, the creation of new beds, and improvements in admission policies were closely related to the surrounding economic conditions, a dependence that is clearly visible whenever a hospital went through an economic crisis. But on the basis of what I have noted above, it would seem that the founding of a hospital, which is an outstanding gesture, and its maintenance even under precarious conditions, in other words the entire structure of the hospital system in its external aspects, were relatively independent of economic factors.

On the other hand, different levels of prosperity may have had indirect effects on the nature of these establishments. As everyone knows by now, the unequal distribution of prosperity in early-modern France resulted in a cultural contrast favoring northern France. Now that is precisely the region where the largest number of hôtels-Dieu, establishments exclusively catering to the sick, were located. Their presence, a most remarkable fact, seems to me to be in part related to the early dissemination of a "modern" mentality, underlaid here by a cultural development that gradually stripped disease of its fateful character and its ascetic value. It appears that at a very early date, and in a somewhat unplanned manner, the task of combating disease was entrusted to the hôtel-Dieu; and one might say that the occasional misuse of this term, which had been quite precise even in the Middle Ages, is as valid an indication as the actual daily functioning of these establishments in northern France. In this manner northern France added one more characteristic to all the others that constituted its modernity, namely, a special system of hospitals, the very system that by the end of the eighteenth century was perceived as a necessary waystation for any medical progress.

Given the variety of establishments known under the name of hospitals, it is understandable that contemporaries could not consider their large number alone as an indication of remarkable development. At most, they felt that their profusion—which usually went hand in hand with mediocrity—was the sign of an archaic situation, of a world left behind by transformations in the welfare system that for a long time were alone considered beneficial. Seen in this manner, the extraordinary concentration of hospitals in Provence, a part of Languedoc, and Roussillon—definitely related to the conjunction of many factors—would be just one more element used to contrast an "uncivilized" France with a "well-policed" one. Finally, and this does not imply any value judgment, certain disparities with respect to national integration might also explain the shadings in the maps of hospitals in southern France and perhaps French Flanders as well. The central government may have hesitated to impose a strict rationalization of local hospital systems on rebellious or recently annexed regions. For whenever this rationalization, which took the form of a wave of *mergers,* was carried out, it generated a disaffection that the authorities were well advised to avoid when it could easily degenerate into festering political opposition.[76]

In the form of hospices or nursing centers, hospitals respond to the fundamental needs of a society trying to deal with illness and old age, which —especially in the past—deprive most people of all resources. Nonetheless, the manner in which human distress is perceived is culturally determined, and hospital establishments are therefore related to more than rational considerations based on numbers and need. In the Ancien Régime, as we have seen, hospitals were clearly related to many factors, many of them acting in covert ways, but undoubtedly always and everywhere, to a greater or lesser extent, with religious considerations playing a particularly important role. A combination of factors can be at work, of course; thus it is the convergence of an advancing urbanization, an intensely experienced religiosity, a baroque temperament, an unusual "sociability," and a certain distance toward the central power that accounts, in Provence, for instance, and to some extent in French Flanders, for the presence of an exceptional number of hospitals. Yet in other areas there was a cruel lack of them. Having learned that hospitals, whatever their density, also represented a phenomenon related to a relatively major population center and that there were no alternative solutions for rural areas,[77] one can well understand why the insufficiency of hospital establishments in relation to the real need of the population gave rise to violent criticism. So violent indeed was this criticism that one is liable to overlook the fact that the presence of a hospital in most towns of over 2,000 inhabitants, with a number of beds only slightly lower than sixty years later (and this despite a rise in population), objectively represented a remarkable phenomenon.

In fact, this is why the members of the specialized Revolutionary committees were particularly interested in the fundamental problem of hospital distribution, trying to establish a rational system by means of an ideal ratio of beds/population and a geographical distribution that would conform to the new administrative organization of France. Such a rationalized system was still not in existence by the middle of the nineteenth century. The committees concerned with beggary and public relief (*Comité de Mendicité* and *Comité de Secours Public*)—and it should be noted that they were heirs to a current of thought preceding the Revolution, to which many of the members had actually contributed—had in fact very accurately pinpointed the main flaws in the system of hospitals. In this manner, the second serious insufficiency they attempted to remedy concerned the shortcomings of a system that was essentially devoted to the care of old age and poverty. They were quick to point out that this could not be dealt with by the hospital. Paralleling a solid organization of medical care delivered in the home or in dispensaries,[78] one therefore sees the first outline of the contemporary hospital, essentially devoted to medical objectives, in the projects of the Legislative and Constituent Assemblies, projects that were informed by intelligence, generosity, and a sense of the possible.[79] For them, utopia would come eventually. A partial solution to all problems would have to wait even longer.

NOTES

1. Jacques Tenon, *Oeuvre manuscrite,* Bibliothèque Nationale, Paris (hereafter B.N.), NAF 22 743, fol. 222.

2. Abbé de Recalde, *Traité sur les abus qui subsistent dans les hôpitaux du royaume et les moyens propres à la réforme afin de rendre l'établissement des maisons de charité utile à l'humanité et glorieux pour la nation* (Paris, 1786), p. 4. In the nineteenth century, de Gasparin, minister of the interior, still wrote in *Rapport au roi sur les hôpitaux, les hospices et les*

maisons de bienfaisance (Paris, 1837), p. 2, that "France does not yield to any other country with respect to the number of its establishments."

3. Tenon, B.N., NAF 22 743, fol. 242.

4. Muriel Joerger, "Les Enquêtes hospitalières au XVIIIe siècle," *Bulletin de la Société française d'histoire des hôpitaux* 31 (1975).

5. Jacques Necker, *De l'administration des finances de la France* (Paris, 1784), vol. 3, ch. 16, p. 176.

6. I am thinking, of course, of Michel Foucault, *Histoire de la folie*, 2nd. ed. (Paris, 1974) [abridged translation by Richard Howard under the title *Madness and Civilization* (New York, 1967)]; also J.-P. Gutton, *La Société et les pauvres: L'Exemple de la généralité de Lyon, 1534-1789* (Paris, 1970); Olwen Huften, *The Poor of Eighteenth Century France, 1750-1789* (Oxford, 1974); Natalie Z. Davis, "Assistance, humanisme et hérésie: Le Cas de Lyon" (1968), reprinted in M. Mollat, ed., *Etudes sur l'histoire de la pauvreté* (Paris, 1974); B. Geremek, "Criminalité, vagabondage, pauperisme: La Marginalité à l'aube des temps modernes," *Revue d'histoire moderne et contemporaine* 21 (July-September 1974): 337-75.

7. In *Naissance de la clinique: Une Archéologie du regard medical*, 2nd ed. (Paris, 1972) [translated by A. H. Sheridan Smith as *Birth of the Clinic* (New York, 1973)], Michel Foucault studies this passage in itself; F. Lebrun, in *Les Hommes et la mort en Anjou aux XVIIe et XVIIIe siècles* (Paris-The Hague, 1971), has occasion to do so within a larger framework.

8. It is impossible to cite all these studies here, but the *Bulletin de la Société des hôpitaux*, ably directed by M. Candille, regularly reports on them in the most conscientious manner.

9. Jacques Tenon, *Mémoires sur les hôpitaux de Paris* (Paris, 1788), p. 1.

10. This committee combined the responsibilities of the committees on begging (*mendicité*) and public health (*salubrité*) of the preceeding Assembly. For this last committee, see L. Ferdinand-Dreyfus, *L'Assistance sous la Législative et la Convention* (Paris, 1905).

11. From the circular launching this survey, which has left very few traces in the archives. Circular 1083 in the departmental archives (hereafter cited as A.D, followed by the name of the department) of Somme, is one example.

12. Jacques Tenon (1724-1816), a renowned surgeon and member of the Académie des Sciences, became known to a wider public when in 1788 he published his *Mémoire sur les hôpitaux de Paris*. His papers, almost all of which were written after that date, are preserved in the Bibliothèque Nationale, Paris. On this subject, see P. Huard, "Les Papiers de J. Tenon," in *Compte rendu du XIX Congrès international d'histoire de la médecine* (Basel, 1964).

13. Actually, the survey of the Committee on Public Relief (*secours public*) did no more than repeat—in the same terms and to the point of irritating those municipalities that had already responded—the survey of the Committee on Begging (*mendicité*), of which many fragments are kept in the departmental archives. The survey of 1791-92 duplicates the preceeding one to such a degree that, to cite one example, the "Tenon list" for Bas-Rhin exactly reproduces the list sent to that department for verification by the Comité de Mendicité (A.D., Bas-Rhin, L 1086), although no trace of a response can be found. Yet we know that the lists of the Comité de Mendicité always needed correction.

14. To begin with, neither of these two surveys was completed, both because time was too short and because of lack of interest on the part of the local authorities. Moreover, it was not possible to include in the lists of the Tenon papers drawn up for a "report on the hospitals of the Republic" prepared by Tenon those responses that arrived later. (See, for example, the extremely faulty Tenon lists for the departments of Gers and Charente-Inférieure and the complete responses prepared by these departments [A.D., Gers, L 427, and Archives nationales, hereafter cited as A.N., F^15 260]).

15. Cf. the text of the circulars launching the survey of the Comité de Mendicité in C. Bloch and A. Tuetey, *Procès-verbaux et rapport du Comité de Mendicité* (Paris, 1911), pp. 244, 251.

16. These figures have been checked against the responses to the surveys by the Revolutionary committees preserved in the departmental archives (series L) or in the National Archives (series F^15). Moreover, I have made a systematic study of all the eighteenth-century hospital surveys prior to the Revolution (A.N., series M, or A.D., series C). Surveys conducted by two intendants after 1750 have been a most important aid in this undertaking (see Manuscript Sources in the bibliography), as have been all the older or recent books and articles about a specific hospital establishment. (Cf. the card catalogue by department of the Bibliothèque de l'Assistance publique in Paris.)

17. *Hôtel-Dieu, maison-Dieu, hôpital général, charité, hospice, maison des pauvres, hôpital*

de charité, hôpital de bienfaisance, . . . hôpital, etc. For this problem of terminology, see C. Bloch, *L'Assistance et l'état en France à la veille de la Révolution* (Paris, 1908), and M. Candille, "Les Mots hôpital et hospices dans la terminologie du XVIIIᵉ siècle," *L'Hôpital et l'aide sociale* (1964).

18. For the fundamental question of spiritual care for hospital inmates, see L. Pérouas, *Le Diocèse de La Rochelle de 1648 à 1724, sociologie et pastorale* (Paris, 1964), p. 395, and Lebrun, *Les Hommes et la Mort en Anjou,* p. 391.

19. Since a recapitulation by J. Tenon (B.N., NAF 22 742, fol. 219) lists the most common designations for hospitals "designed to provide relief in the home," it was easy to eliminate these institutions. Except where more precise information concerning them was available, "charitable foundations," which often simply provided relief to the poor, were also eliminated.

20. The following description, being meant only to prepare the reader for arguments to be developed later, is reduced to a strict minimum. Presenting it in this manner considerably impoverishes the content of an institution whose implications were very widespread indeed.

21. Tenon indignantly noted that the word "incurable" was used "for anyone who is not cured in six months in a hospital where fever and injuries are treated. Nothing is less proven than such an assertion" (B.N., NAF 22 743).

22. For the transformation of general hospitals into hospices, despite a set of rules that by the eighteenth century "were deeply rooted in a tradition of confinement," see J. P. Gutton, *L'Etat et la mendicité dans la première moitié du XVIIIᵉ siècle: Auvergne, Beaujolais, Forez, Lyonnais* (Centre d'Etudes Forésiennes, 1973), p. 26. Cf. also C. Paultre, *De la répression de la mendicité et du vagabondage en France sous l'Ancien Régime* (Paris, 1906).

23. See, among many others, the following request for funds for the general hospital of Sedan (A.N., F¹⁵ 334), where "nineteen-twentieths of the inmates are workers in the cloth manufacturing trade who, reduced to indigence when work is lacking or when illness and old age overcome them, can only turn to this house as a resource for themselves and their children."

24. J. Tenon—in whose writings we often see compassion shining through statements of fact—was to give beautiful expression to the sadness and astonishment the general hospital provoked in him: "One wonders why there has to be this neglect of basic needs, this crushing of childhood, of the aged, and of the infirm" (B.N., NAF 22 743).

25. For *many* reasons, the use of this source—especially for the end of the eighteenth century—is questionable; but what else could give us as exhaustive and, when all is said and done, accurate data? Thanks to the indications of the Laboratoire de Cartographie, directed by J. Mallet, whom I wish to thank here, along with his staff, I was able to adjust the limits of the departments and thereby modify the population figures in order to recreate, more or less accurately, the situation of 1791. In examining individual towns I have always made use of the most recent studies.

26. All of the mathematical and statistical calculations are due to M. Demonet, whose patience and kindness I gratefully acknowledge.

27. Checks against other sources have almost always led to subtractions rather than additions.

28. In 1847, Vaucluse and Bouches-du-Rhône (constituting *roughly* the department of Bouches-du-Rhône of 1792) were first and fourth, respectively; Var was third; Seine-et-Oise fifth; Seine-et-Marne ninth.

29. M. Agulhon, *Pénitents et francs-maçons de l'ancienne Provence* (Paris, 1968), p. 32; M. Vovelle, *Piété baroque et déchristianisation* (Paris, 1974). Although he points out that these institutions were "sometimes rather humble," Vovelle did find hospitals in almost half of the 190 villages he studied.

30. Beds were doubled and tripled in the hôtels-Dieu of Paris, Tours (F¹⁵ 227), and Limoges (F¹⁵ 228-1). There are innumerable testimonies about the general hospitals, where "the number of poor is unlimited." At Marseilles, for instance, the number of beds rose fourfold from one survey to the next (A.D., Bouches-du-Rhône, R 4196).

31. His data were used for the report by Watteville: *Rapport à monsieur le ministre de l'Intérieur sur l'administration des hôpitaux et des hospices* (Paris, 1851). This report makes a distinction between the sick and the old, a distinction that does not appear in the *Statistique générale de la France* until 1853.

32. This assertion is based on a calculation too long to be reproduced here. It takes into account the existence of 133 hospitals with less than ten beds in 1847, by contrast with 595 such hospitals at the end of the eighteenth century.

33. The data concerning the contemporary period (1973, to be exact) are taken from the publications of the Ministry of Health, *Santé, sécurité sociale, statistiques et commentaires* (1975), no. 4. vol. A; *Statistiques annuelles des hôpitaux publiées* (1975), no. 4, vol. B. See also *Recensement des établissements d'hospitalisation privés*, a joint publication of the Ministry of Health and the Ministry of Labor. In order to obtain the findings presented in the text, I have combined the figures of the Department of Public Welfare with those of the private sector.

34. Jean-Pierre Goubert and F. Lebrun, "Médecins et chirurgiens dans la société française du XVIIIe siècle," *Medicina, economia e società nell'esperienza statica*, Congresso internationale (Pavia, 1973); J.-C. Perrot, *Genèse d'une ville moderne: Caen au XVIIIe siècle* (Paris, 1975), 2: 283. Small hôtels-Dieu made do with surgeons, and so, often, did the large ones, because of the lack of interest of many physicians. The physicians' attitude toward the hospital, which they treated with "a kind of indifference" (Iberti, *Réflexions sur les hôpitaux* [Paris, 1788]), would deserve a close analysis.

35. Compare the following figures: the number of beds in the forty-two departments where more than 70 percent of the establishments (the aggregate total is 86.70 percent) indicated their capacity was 32,596. By 1837, it had risen to 44,002 units in these same departments, although all establishments were counted.

36. For a very long time—since this was still the case under the Second Empire (cf. *Situation administrative et financière des hôpitaux de l'Empire*, published under the direction of de Lurieu [Paris, 1869], 1: xi)—hospital administrators did not "fix" a precise number of beds strictly reserved for the sick in every "mixed" establishment. For this reason one is surprised that Watteville in his report of 1847 does not mention any problem and unequivocally states the respective number of beds for the sick and for the inmates of hospices.

37. R. Bridgman, *L'Hôpital et la cité* (Paris, 1965), p. 108, examines this index furnished by Clavareau, *Mémoires sur les hôpitaux civils de Paris* (Paris, 1805), p. 231.

38. The "censuses of the hospital population" annually called for by Necker beginning in 1778, a source available for a period of ten years and a third of France's *généralités*, show that on 1 January there were always as many individuals as there were beds (cf. Joerger, "Les Enquêtes hospitalières"). Moreover, it should also be noted that these censuses very faithfully reflect the differences among the three types of hospital treated here, for the mortality of the permanent inmates shows a very distinct pattern.

39. That terror was often invoked by the subdelegates or by a parish priest to demonstrate to the detractors of the hospital, who associated it with laziness, that one "did not go there as if it were a pleasure party" (Poyet, *Mémoire sur la nécessité de transférer l'hôtel-Dieu* [Paris, 1785]). See the statements cited by A. Poitrineau, *La Vie rurale en basse Auvergne au XVIIIe siècle, 1726-1789* (Paris, 1965), 2: 100.

40. Report of the commissioners charged with examining the project for the new hôtel-Dieu by the Académie des Sciences (*Régistre de l'Académie des Sciences*, 22 November 1786, p. 109).

41. Did the profession go so far as to think that hospitals, while conferring experience, might also serve for experimentation? Aikin, in *Réflexions sur les hôpitaux* (French translation, 1787), p. 75, rejects this notion, but such writings as *Essai sur les établissements nécessaires et les moins dispendieux pour rendre le service des malades dans les hôpitaux vraiment utile à l'humanité* (Paris, 1787), p. 11, by a certain Dulaurens, and *Moyens de rendre les hôpitaux plus utiles à la nation* (Paris, 1787), pp. 169 ff., by a certain Chambon de Monteaux, are disturbing. This ambiguity was, of course, very well perceived by Foucault in *Birth of the Clinic*.

42. I had already cited this quote from Tenon (B.N., NAF 22 743) in my article "Les Enquêtes hospitalières," for it very clearly sums up its author's thinking and the entire set of problems raised by the question of hospitals in the late eighteenth century. This quote, incidentally, also serves as the title of the latest work published under the direction of Michel Foucault, *Les Machines à guérir* (Paris, 1977), which was published as I was correcting the proofs of the present article. Now that it is available, the reader is advised to use this collective work, which shows the medicalization of the hospital by means of precise facts.

43. This is the very foundation of Tenon's thinking, running through all of his published work. Cf. also Cabanis, "Observations sur les hôpitaux" (1790) in *Oeuvres complètes* (1956). Yet the hospital, even the hospital for the sick, had its fierce detractors, among whom Dupont de Nemours, with his *Idées sur les secours à donner* (Paris, 1786), is the most famous. The Comité de Mendicité, which on this point disagreed fundamentally with both the Comité de Salubrité of the same Assembly and the Comité des Secours Publics established by the

Legislative Assembly, reflects the tendency of those who wanted the sick to be cared for at home.

44. See map no. 1 in A. d'Angeville, *Essai sur la statistique de la population française, 1836* (Paris, 1969). Aside from Moselle and Bouches-du-Rhône, which were more highly populated in 1831 than in 1806, it is very similar to the approximate map I had drawn up as a control measure on the basis of the census of 1806.

45. Bouches-du-Rhône, Var, and Hautes-Alpes, as well as Seine-et-Oise and Seine-et-Marne.

46. This ratio (0.68) is lower than the ratio cited above (0.75) because I based my statistical calculations on the census of 1806, which gives a population figure of 28,644,463 rather than the 26,000,000 used to obtain the ratio of 0.75. At the departmental level these distortions are not as great and do not warp the general reading.

47. Forty-two rather than forty-three, for I have excluded from this calculation the department of Seine, given the manner in which its enormous traditional hospital capacity weights the statistics. In fact, this department is often excluded from certain calculations even today to avoid skewing the averages.

48. Yet if this remark is to assume general validity, a systematic study must be carried out. Caen, for example, has a ratio of 15.05 and Nantes of 9.58.

49. The expression was coined by X. Leclainche and A. Gardie, *Enquête hospitalière générale* (Paris, 1954).

50. This problem was treated extensively by Bridgman, *L'Hôpital et la cité*. Studying the contemporary period, Bridgman found that the situation was largely rooted in the past until about twenty years ago. He concluded that there was a clear correlation between patterns of settlement and a small number of hospitals.

51. For the percentage of urban population and its cartographic representation, see R. Le Mee, "Population agglomérée et population éparse au début du XIXe siècle," *Annales de démographie historique* (1971): 494.

52. See the resumé of the papers of the Académie de Châlons, *Les Moyens de détruire la mendicité en France en rendant les mendiants utiles à l'Etat sans les rendre malheureux* (Châlons-Paris, 1780). These are resumés of papers competing for the prize of the Académie des Sciences, Arts et Belles Lettres of Châlons-sur-Marne in 1777. See also the projects for hospital reform enumerated in n. 79, below.

53. In the name of the imperatives of urban policy, the profitability of installations, and a rationality partly warranted by the modern means of transportation.

54. Actually, the contrast between the "dechristianized" town and the fervent countryside dates only from the end of the eighteenth and especially the nineteenth centuries.

55. One must start with the end of the Middle Ages, when there were "very few villages without a little house for taking care of the sick" (M. Mollat, *Etude sur l'histoire de la pauvreté* [Paris, 1974], p. 5), and look at maps of a region at the end of the fifteenth and in the eighteenth century in Gutton, *La Société et les pauvres,* pp. 280, 476. See also J. Jenny, "Les Oeuvres de charité et les institutions hospitalières dans le diocèse de Bourges, XVIIe-XVIIIe siècles," *32e Congrès de la Fédération des sociétés savantes du Centre* (Guéret, 1972); T. J. Schmitt, *L'Assistance dans l'archidiacôné d'Autun de 1650 à 1750* (Autun, 1957); Lebrun, *Les Hommes et la mort en Anjon.*

56. Geremek, "Criminalité," and Davis, "Assistance, humanisme et hérésie"; also J. Delumeau, *La Civilisation de la Renaissance* (Paris, 1967), who stresses a notion that is too often overlooked when the coercive urban mentality is condemned, namely, the extreme "vulnerability" of the old city.

57. Cf. Paultre, *De la répression,* as well as the astonishing founding of the general hospital of Bourges described by Jenny in "Les Oeuvres de charité."

58. Cf. M. Agulhon, "La Notion de village en Provence," *Actes du congrès des sociétés savantes de Nice* (Nice, 1965).

59. At Pontoise or Senlis, for example.

60. Cf. Vovelle, *Piété baroque,* chap. 6.

61. Cf. F. Dissart, "La Réforme des maladreries et hôpitaux au XVIIe siècle," (Thesis in law, University of Paris, 1938). In 1752, upon completion of one survey, the intendants were asked to submit an additional report about possible mergers within their *généralités* (cf. Joerger, "Les Enquêtes hospitalières").

62. In a letter to the archbishop of Toulouse (A.N., F^{15} 138), informing him that a survey of hopitals had been launched.

63. Pérouas, *Le Diocèse de La Rochelle,* p. 397, shows the progressive spread of the

enthusiasm for founding hospitals from the town to the "rural countryside." Vovelle, in *Piété baroque*, p. 253, evokes "the village hospital . . . constantly spreading throughout the eighteenth century."

64. Cf. the reactions of a certain Colombier, an excellent administrator and expert in all problems connected with hospitals, a figure to whom modern historiography does not pay enough attention. Having close ties to Necker, who had created the position of *inspecteur général des hôpitaux* for him, Colombier represents the attitudes of the governing elites. Significantly, he advocated the restoration of a six-bed hospital at Coursan (A.N., F[15] 138) and felt that the tendency to let small hospitals in Hainaut "fall into ruins" was "vicious" (A.N., F[15] 228-1). Cf. also J. D. Gallot, *Extrait d'un mémoire sur les maladies populaires avec les moyens de soulagements publics pour les pauvres de la campagne* (Paris, 1787).

65. Howard, *Etat des prisons et des hôpitaux*, French trans. (Paris, 1788), 1: 352. visiting the two men's hospitals at Lille, Howard noted: "When a new patient comes in, . . . one of the sisters . . . washes his feet, dries them, and kisses one of them"; a gesture that is obviously taken from the Gospel.

66. Pérouas, *Le Diocèse de La Rochelle*, p. 342. In emphasizing the charitable achievements of the Protestants, Pérouas depicts a "situation that demanded action." For somewhat different reasons, this was also true with respect to the *"petites écoles;"* cf. Mireille Laget, "Petites écoles en Languedoc au XVIIIe siècle," *Annales, E.S.C.* 26 (November-December 1971): 1398.

67. J. Ferté, *La Vie religieuse dans les campagnes parisiennes, 1622-25* (Paris, 1962).

68. Cf. the map "Extension du jansénisme richériste" in E. Préclin, *Les Jansénistes au XVIIIe siècle* (Paris, 1929), p. 124.

69. R. Taverneau, *Le Jansénisme en Lorraine* (Paris, 1962), and P. Chaunu, "Jansénisme et frontière de catholicité," *Revue Historique* 227 (January-March 1962): 115-38.

70. In the eighteenth century it was commonplace to establish a relation of cause and effect between the poverty of Spain and Italy and the profusion there of hospitals, which were accused of fostering laziness.

71. In the case of the Netherlands, the high population density is to some extent sufficient to account for the great number of hospitals. Nonetheless, the fact that it was possible to establish enough institutions to satisfy such intense demand might be worth explaining in greater depth.

72. In *Piété baroque*, p. 246, Vovelle also speaks of the "ambiguity of the charitable gesture in the baroque period," a time when "poor people for the solemn funerals of notables were supplied by the hospitals, since they could no longer be found in the streets."

73. Review of M. Agulhon, *La Sociabilité méridionale*, by M. Vovelle, in *Revue de l'histoire de l'Eglise de France* (1967).

74. For the brotherhoods engaged in managing hospital foundations, see Agulhon, *Pénitents et francs-maçons*, p. 32.

75. See the "famous map" (P. Chaunu's expression) siting these "faculties" in P. de Dainville, "Un Dénombrement inédit au XVIIIe siècle: L'Enquête du contrôleur général Orry," *Population* 7 (January-March 1952): 49-68. This map is corroborated by later studies (see E. Le Roy Ladurie, introduction to d'Angeville, *Essai sur la statistique*, pp. xviii-xix.

76. In any case, the long report by the intendant of Roussillon concerning possible mergers (1752, Boullogne survey, A.D., Pyrénées-Orientales, C 1133) did not lead to any change whatsoever: in 1785 the hospitals mentioned by him were still there. Because of unending litigation, the general hospital of Perpignan was never able to obtain certain "mergers," even though they had been officially decided upon in the second half of the eighteenth century.

77. Even if there was a physician or a surgeon not too far away in a small town, "they do not come out here free of charge" (*Cahier* of Allerey, cited in P. de Saint-Jacob, *Les Paysans de la Bourgogne du nord au dernier siècle de l'Ancien Régime* [Paris, 1960], p. 545). Poitrineau, in *La Vie rurale*, also stresses the deprivation of the rural population caused by the high cost of medical care.

78. The word—imported from England—and the institution already existed. It was hoped that the latter could be extended in order to free more hospital beds.

79. The projects of the Comité de Mendicité are to be found in the committee's report no. 4 (Bloch and Tuetey, *Procès-verbaux*); those of the various comités de secours public were outlined in the report of deputy Bernard, "Rapport au nom du Comité de Secours Public sur les secours à donner aux indigents," *Archives parlementaires* (1792), and in Tenon's unfinished "Discours sur les hôpitaux civils de la République," B.N. NAF 22 743.

SOURCES AND BIBLIOGRAPHY

Manuscript Sources

FONDS TENON

Concerning hospitals, the Tenon Papers of the Bibliothèque Nationale contain several incomplete lists and a large number of outlines of breakdowns or unfinished totals. Aside from these, the most complete recapitulations (which I have used here) are to be found under the following call numbers:

— NAF 22 742, fol. 49: "Hôpitaux de France distribués par départements."

— NAF 22 743, fol. 219: "Rapports sur les hôpitaux civils de la République," which includes a breakdown of hospitals into four categories, "les hôpitaux de valides," "les hôpitaux de malades," "les établissements pour secourir à domicile," and "les maisons contre la fragilité de la jeunesse."

— NAF 22 747, fol. 1: "Table des établissements par catégorie particulière distribués par ordre alphabétique avec indication de la ville ou du département"; fol. 39: "Récapitulation du nombre et de la nature des hôpitaux en France."

— NAF 22 750: The catalogue as a whole includes a "dénombrement des hôpitaux de France rassemblés par J. Tenon."

(N.B.: Corsica, which was unable to send in its response, is excluded from these data. So is the department of Seine, although no explanation is given for this lacuna. For the latter department, I have used J. Tenon, *Mémoire sur les hôpitaux de Paris* [Paris, 1788] and such information as can be found in the Archives nationales.)

MANUSCRIPTS

"Mémoires de 1766 sur la généralité de Tours" (Bibliothèque municipale of Château-Gontier); De Balainvilliers, "Mémoires sur le Languedoc" (1788) (Bibliothèque municipale of Montpellier, fonds Languedoc no. 15). I have used a copy of volume 3, devoted to hospitals and charity houses, which can be found at the Bibliothèque de l'Assistance publique [welfare department] of Paris.

CENSUS OF 1806

A. N. F^{20} 30 and 33; Service historique de l'armée, Vincennes: The call numbers of these *mémoires* and *reconnaissances* are 1118-19. (For the most part, I have used the microfilms very kindly lent to me by A. Bergeron.)

NATIONAL ARCHIVES

Series M 673-76; Series F^{15} 226-30, 235, 249, 251-55, 260-71, 282, 310, 318, 320.

DEPARTMENTAL ARCHIVES

Aisne C 665-66, L 1516; Ariège 1 C 184; Bouches-du-Rhône C 3215, 4196, L 494, 856-59, 1488-91; Calvados C 1044; Cher C 41, 150-65; Côte-d'Or C 376-79; Doubs, C 121-23, 1 and 2; Drôme L 621; Gers C 333, L 427; Gironde C 1104-7, C supplement 3664; Hérault C 5956; Ille-et-Vilaine C 1293; Indre L 1250; Loir-et-Cher L 756; Marne C 1940; Haute-Marne C 36,

84 205; Meurthe-et-Moselle C 339; Morbihan L 885; Nord L 5286, 5287, 5979; Orne C 273, 274; Puy-de-Dôme, C 927-38, 1438-47; Pyrénées-Orientales C 1133, 1138; Bas-Rhin C 228, L 1250, 646, 647; Rhône C 162, 166-69; Seine-inférieure C 995-98; Somme L 427, 1083.

APPENDIX 1

Correlation between the Number of Hospitals and the Number of Beds with the Population Figure

The Correlation Index

For hospitals as well as beds there was a correlation, provided that the index obtained was higher than 0.39. To be exact, in that case there was less than one chance in 100 that no correlation existed. The index was 0.71 for hospitals and 0.66 for beds.

Distribution of the Indices

Table 6.1—Average Weighted Spread

	Number of Departments Considered	Average Weighted Spread	Highest Index	Lowest Index	Weighted Average
Hospitals	82	0.61	3.09	0.42	0.68
	77	0.35	1.42	0.30	0.60
	55	0.34	1.42	0.30	0.56
Beds	42	0.67	7.24	0.70	2.19

Note: 82 departments: France minus Corsica
77 departments:France minus Provence (Var, Bouches-du-Rhône, Basses-Alpes), Seine-et-Marne, and Seine-et-Oise
55 departments: all of the departments where it was possible to verify more than 70 percent of the establishments
42 departments: all of the departments (except Seine) that furnished the number of beds for more than 70 percent of their establishments

Table 6.2—Breakdown of Indices

	Number of Departments Considered	Percentage of Indices Used	Lowest Value	Highest Value	Weighted Average
Hospitals	82	50	0.45	0.74	0.68
	77	50	0.44	0.73	0.60
	55	50	0.41	0.67	0.56
Beds	42	50	1.14	2.43	2.19

Note: see table 6.1 note, above

APPENDIX 2

Numerical Distribution of Hospitals and Hospital Beds and Ranking of All Departments

Table 6.3 – Numerical Distribution of Hospitals and Hospital Beds and Ranking of All Departments

Department	Total Number of Hospitals	Level of Verification (%)	Rank of Department by Total Number of Hospitals	Index of Hospitals per 10,000 Inhabitants	Index of Beds per 1,000 Inhabitants
Ain	18	94	43	0.59	2.99
Aisne	26	88	24	0.58	1.59
Allier	18	78	43	0.69	1.29
Basses-Alpes	47	43	7	3.09	–
Hautes-Alpes	7	71	82	0.56	0.96
Ardèche	13	77	64	0.44	–
Ardennes	13	67	64	0.47	–
Ariège	15	87	57	0.67	0.76
Aube	20	53	40	0.85	–
Aude	14	57	62	0.58	–
Aveyron	21	67	35	0.63	–
Bouches-du-Rhône	91	68	1	1.91	3.47
Calvados	21	78	27	0.41	0.95
Cantal	10	100	76	0.39	0.76
Charente	13	100	64	0.39	1.74
Charente inférieure	15	80	57	0.36	2.28
Cher	18	94	43	0.78	2.24
Corrèze	14	83	64	0.51	2.24
Côte-d'Or	23	86	28	0.64	3.10
Côtes-du-Nord	16	100	55	0.30	1.35
Creuse	10	100	76	0.44	0.92
Dordogne	23	100	28	0.54	0.73
Doubs	11	82	74	0.48	3.23
Drôme	36	74	11	1.42	–
Eure	31	76	17	0.73	1.30
Eure-et-Loire	31	68	17	1.16	–

Gard	22	82	33	0.33	2.38
Haute-Garonne	39	36	8	0.68	—
Gers	17	82	49	1.06	—
Gironde	21	48	35	0.57	—
Hérault	34	88	13	0.40	4.58
Ille-et-Vilaine	21	81	35	1.13	—
Indre	15	93	57	0.41	0.76
Indre-et-Loire	18	83	43	0.73	—
Isère	39	67	8	0.65	—
Jura	13	83	71	0.82	1.38
Landes	12	100	64	0.93	—
Loir-et-Cher	13	92	64	0.54	1.97
Haute-Loire	17	100	49	0.60	2.69
Loire inférieure	17	100	49	0.63	2.68
Loiret	35	43	12	0.41	—
Lot	17	60	49	1.22	—
Lot-et-Garonne	19	100	42	0.46	0.70
Lozère	9	89	80	0.58	1.91
Maine-et-Loire	34	59	13	0.62	—
Manche	21	81	35	0.84	2.34
Marne	23	78	28	0.36	4.84
Haute-Marne	12	83	72	0.50	1.50
Mayenne	14	64	62	0.76	—
Meurthe	31	77	17	0.42	—
Meuse	18	41	43	0.84	—
Morbihan	15	100	57	0.63	1.92
Moselle	23	65	28	0.37	—
Nièvre	15	80	57	0.62	1.83
Nord	62	84	3	0.73	—
Oise	31	47	17	0.83	—
Orne	17	71	49	0.40	1.50
Pas-de-Calais	34	44	13	0.59	—
Puy-de-Dôme	30	86	21	0.55	2.35
Basses-Pyrénées	11	70	74	0.38	—
Hautes-Pyrénées	9	56	80	0.45	—
Pyrénées-Orientales	13	100	64	1.02	3.07
Bas-Rhin	21	62	35	0.41	—
Haut-Rhin	20	100	40	0.62	—

Table 6.3 (continued)

Department	Total Number of Hospitals	Level of Verification (%)	Rank of Department by Total Number of Hospitals	Index of Hospitals per 10,000 Inhabitants	Index of Beds per 1,000 Inhabitants
Rhône-et-Loire	23	100	28	0.34	7.24
Saône	10	76	76	0.33	0.81
Saône-et-Loire	24	96	26	0.50	2.14
Sarthe	39	38	8	0.95	—
Seine	50	100	5	0.74	—
Seine inférieure	32	61	16	0.49	—
Seine-et-Marne	49	51	6	1.61	—
Seine-et-Oise	59	49	4	1.36	—
Deux-Sèvres	17	53	49	0.66	—
Somme	30	70	21	0.60	1.75
Tarn	22	67	33	0.70	—
Var	87	67	2	3.07	—
Vendée	10	70	76	0.37	1.14
Vienne	16	67	55	0.63	2.43
Haute-Vienne	18	65	43	0.74	—
Vosges	17	82	49	0.50	0.87
Yonne	27	70	23	0.82	1.18

7
Childbirth in Seventeenth- and Eighteenth-Century France: Obstetrical Practices and Collective Attitudes

Mireille Laget

Does childbirth lie beyond the scope of history? Is the act of giving birth fixed in its most inward aspects? Is it subject to a set of immutable external rituals permanently present in time and geographical space, namely, the ritual of a physiological process, the ritual of suffering experienced in the company of women, and the ritual surrounding a child's first breath?[1] In the same manner as death, as all important moments in the life of women and men, the act of giving birth revolves upon specific social and cultural pressures that are extremely slow to change. Trying to show the emotions, taboos, or techniques of French society in the Ancien Régime may well amount to ascertaining their continued existence in our own mental universe.

I therefore feel that I cannot limit my investigation to a set chronological framework or to the specialist's perspective. In saying this, I am expressing my uneasiness at trying to shed light on a moment in life that we can only understand by means of a number of approaches, namely, those of the psychologist, the ethnographer, the woman in childbirth, and the average person. For in fact the greatest difficulty for anyone who tries to understand is the total lack of firsthand testimony. To be sure, the famous obstetricians of the seventeenth and eighteenth centuries have described their "parturients" and displayed their miraculous interventions. But did they ever question the women in childbirth? What ethnologist can systematically witness a birth to which he is a stranger? Documents only recite the facts. By the same token,

Annales, E.S.C. 32 (September-October 1977: 958-92. Translated by Elborg Forster.

the phenomena that we assume to be immutable (apprehension and pain, for instance) can be neither certified nor quantified. Childbirth as an ineluctable reality does indeed lie beyond the scope of historical mutations, but also beyond the ken of the historian who lacks the proper tools and works in isolation. The few pages that follow can only outline some analyses whose perspectives, limits, and sources remain to be refined.

Trying to outline a certain number of themes for research in the area of childbirth in the seventeenth and eighteenth centuries is to go beyond historical documentation. Certain perspectives can barely be touched upon, in particular, the data of historical demography (systematic calculations of infant mortality and mortality in childbirth by long series still remain to be carried out), the medical history of the techniques of intervention in childbirth, the chances at birth of the child (was it wanted or rejected? what permitted it to live or to survive?). This last theme may in the future lead to a comprehensive comparative study based on already existing studies on the beginnings of contraception, illegitimate births, infanticide, and the abandonment of children.[2] Within the framework of a more restricted essay, and on the basis of original documents, it is possible to show the attitudes of men and women more or less closely involved with a birth, certain deeply engrained modes of thinking, and the slowness with which these changed.

For Languedoc, the documentary sources are considerable. There are manuals or catechisms on the art of midwifery published in Paris or in the provinces from the time of Henry IV until the Revolution. They can be found in local public and private libraries, especially in the library of the Faculty of Medicine of Montpellier. There are also pamphlets distributed by the Estates [of Languedoc] containing advice to midwives and mothers and criticizing the ignorance of matrons and obstetricians. In the departmental archives of Hérault, a series of learned papers read before the Faculty of Medicine deal with obstetrical difficulties, miraculous or monstrous births, and the resuscitation of newborn infants. A number of bundles in series G contain judicial proceedings against Protestant midwives or notorious abortionists. In municipal series, the minutes of town council meetings or scattered papers contain information about the swearing-in of midwives and the formal approval of the bishop. For the revolutionary era, the opening of a school of midwifery, independent of the Faculty of Medicine and the School of Surgery, is the subject of several bundles in series M (organization, examinations, certification). Finally, we can use the various surveys of the episcopal records, the records concerning practicing midwives of the intendancy and later the prefect's office. Attached to these surveys is an enormous amount of correspondence between the local authorities and the subdelegates. To be sure, the sheer number of documents is not proportionate to their importance for the subject. Nonetheless, they raise certain questions concerning the practices and patterns of behavior connected with childbirth, for, to a greater or lesser extent, these were characteristic of Ancien Régime society. Thus, one would like to know whether social and cultural traditions, modesty, and taboos weighed more heavily on this society than on others or whether one should view the struggle against collective ignorance, prejudice, and indecency waged by the royal power and the medical profession as proof that in the eighteenth century an elite was able to overthrow the most deeply engrained patterns of behavior and to create new patterns within the realm of realism and experience.

Confinements in Shame and Resignation

The social and cultural legacy of a civilization crystallizes around the great moments of life in a complex set of attitudes and fantasies. Childbirth is a unique moment, repeated over and over in the life of a people, "the best opportunity to seize the manner in which culture integrates the crucial natural phenomena into a symbolic network."[3]

In the society of the Ancien Régime, more perhaps than in others, the weight of constraints burdening the conception of a child conferred a stamp of resignation upon motherhood. Ethnologists make much of the "pride in the state of pregnancy" among the most diverse peoples and observe a glorification of the pregnant woman.[4] French women during the reigns of Louis XIV or Louis XV experienced this pride only fleetingly or in a diffuse manner, and only when their lives were not too hard and their bodies not too exhausted. They knew little about pregnancy and usually experienced it as a hardship. In the textbooks devoted to "pregnant and newly delivered women" the woman who expected a child was considered to be a sick person. "Generation" and the period of gestation were treated briefly, in a few pages at most. In the most advanced treatise published in the seventeenth century, François Mauriceau, at one time provost of the master surgeons' guild of the city of Paris, exhibits very primitive notions of genetics and embryology.[5] One of the areas in which the obstetricians made no progress was the question of fertilization; they wondered what kind of seed women secreted. As late as 1796, the great Baudeloque still presented ovulation as a mere hypothesis.[6] From one of these great masters to the other, no notion had really evolved, and J.-N. Biraben justly charges certain of the minor works with crass ignorance.[7]

The same Mauriceau, a great authority in the reign of Louis XIV, published a series of sketches showing the comparative size of the fetus at several stages of pregnancy, showing a child as perfectly formed at one day as at three months, the only difference being its size (see fig. 7.1). In the manual of 1694 by Philippe Peu, first physician to the queen,[8] four plates show the various fetal positions and the possible twists of the umbilical cord, a rare effort at concrete illustration. Here the unborn child assumes the features, the relief, and the posture of a little fresco angel (figs. 7.2 and 7.3). Seventy-five years later the engraver Jean-Christophe Le Ben illustrated Madame Le Boursier Du Coudray's book.[9] Showing the anatomy of the pelvis and the uterus, he

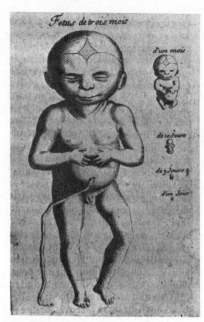

Figure 7.1. Illustration from François Mauriceau, *Traité des maladies des femmes grosses et de celles qui sont accouchées*

depicted a sitting fetus, awaiting the hour of its birth in a pose of patient boredom (fig. 7.4). These works invariably describe only the discomforts of pregnancy implicit in medical prescriptions and moralizing advice.

Was this ignorance fortuitous? Or did it stem not so much from ineptness and lack of technical skill as from fear—fear of everything pertaining to the sexual organs and to reproduction? Throughout the obstetrical literature, one senses an unwillingness to perform an autopsy when a woman died in the early stages of the pregnancy, and one also senses that vaginal examinations were rare, at least before the onset of labor. The few illustrations showing the exterior female anatomy expressly refer to the "shameful parts."[10] Women knew nothing about themselves and did not want to know anything. This attitude is at the core of the ignorance and the age-old psychological block that stood in the way of any realistic contraceptive measures. Steeped in the spirit of religion, this society considered large families a blessing from heaven, while the spacing of births aroused suspicion. There is no doubt that more than one parish priest tried to find out the intimate facts about families in which the mother no longer conceived. For centuries, any contraceptive practice was a "baneful secret" that gave rise to feelings of guilt in couples. A number of modern studies, which I have cited above, have shown the pressure exerted by these taboos[11] and the appearance in the eighteenth century of a brand of French Malthusianism.

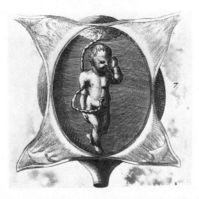

Figure 7.2. Illustration from Philippe Peu, *La Pratique des accouchements*

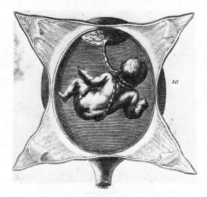

Figure 7.3. Illustration from Philippe Peu, *La Pratique des accouchements*

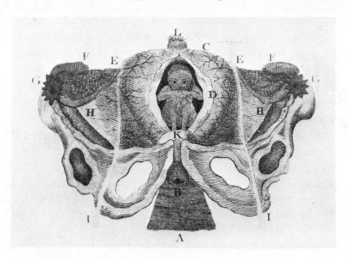

Figure 7.4. Illustration from Mme. Le Boursier du Coudray, *Abrégé de l'art des accouchements*

Among those who began to assert their independence vis-à-vis the Church, were concerned about their children's future, and were more clearly aware of the burden entailed by raising a family,[12] there may well have been radiant mothers corresponding to the images of triumph pictured on the covers of most of the catechisms of midwifery (where the mother appears as a fruitful and exalted Demeter). But in the mass of nameless families the woman was incapable of separating copulation from "generation." She was beyond ignorance, in the realm of the "unthinkable."[13] She was submissive, "illiterate and treated harshly,"[14] in Languedoc and most probably elsewhere; she was worn out by many confinements and sometimes by service as a wetnurse; and she was treated with contempt if she was indigent.[15] She lived through her time of waiting in a state of exhaustion or anxiety. I am speaking here of the exhaustion resulting from pregnancies and miscarriages repeated very year or two, as well as of the anxiety of women who were pregnant outside the social norms. Women in their forties had been unable to avoid ten or twelve pregnancies, even by means of late marriage or abstinence.[16] By the end of their fertile years, they were at the threshold of old age, often suffering the incurable consequences of poorly handled confinements. As for the women whose children were illegitimate, the disapproval of society made them into hunted creatures who tried to hide their pregnancy or to "kill their fruit." Servant girls seduced by their masters, girls impregnated by passing strangers or soldiers, rarely consenting but always accused, they appear more and more frequently on the lists of the parish registers in the course of the eighteenth century. The family rejected them. Public opinion condemned them and obliged them to reveal their secret by all kinds of judicial and psychological means: their declaration of pregnancy was to be made public from the pulpit (although this regulation was often overlooked, especially in rural areas);[17] they were asked to state the father's name, which was extorted "in the last throes of labor"; depositions of midwives and obstetricians were taken. Philippe Ariès has spoken of a "civilization of secrecy." These pregnant women learned to simulate from fear or from poverty. Nicolas Puzos showed how difficult it was to ascertain the pregnancy of a girl who did not want to admit it or of a wetnurse who was afraid that she would have to give up a child who supplemented her family's income.[18] These women would simulate a fit of coughing in order to contract their muscles and keep the child from moving or assert that they suffered from dropsy. The glory of motherhood, though still sung in church, had ceased to be a moral, religious, and artistic ideal.

Contrasting the attitude of primitive peoples, who make the pregnant woman into a sacred object, and the attitude of Western societies, B. Malinowski writes, "In Western societies, pregnancy is considered a burden and a detrimental state; in the upper and middle classes it constitutes a source of embarassment and inconvenience and leads to a temporary interruption of the normal social life."[19] One must be very careful not to attribute the mentality of today's women to women who lived two centuries ago. If one of the objectives of the present study is to show the continued existence of certain patterns of behavior, no purpose is served by projecting our own sensibilities. It is important to rediscover, as certain historians of death such as François Lebrun or Michel Vovelle have done, the emotional universe of men and women of the past. Their feelings of duty accomplished, the permanent climate of insecurity, and their familiarity with hunger, suffering, and early death gave the women of this old society a kind of serenity in the face of their own and their children's destiny.

The subject of the death of the fetus, as well as that of the death of the mother, will be broached later. But in order to understand how a woman experienced the birth of her child, one must recall the frequency of stillbirths and the toleration of infanticide, at least until the end of the seventeenth century. Was the newborn valued as a person? Several historians have analyzed the contradiction perpetuated by the Christian moral code, which made procreation an obligation but also demanded that every child be treated well.[20] The smothering of children in their mothers' or wetnurses' beds was often not accidental. Physicians decried it, and the religious authorities often expressed their concern about it. The following text, one among many, is taken from François Mauriceau's treatise (1668):

Concerning several children smothered by their wetnurses who went to sleep on them while giving them the breast.

On 15 February I delivered a woman of a very beautiful child which unhappily was smothered the next day by its wetnurse who had gone to sleep on this poor child. . . . Since then I have seen five or six other newborn infants as unhappily smothered by their wetnurses who had gone to sleep on them in the same manner while nursing them. These baneful examples point to the need for taking care in a matter of such great importance. Wetnurses must therefore always put their nurseling down separately in a cradle and must never nurse it during the night unless they are quite awake; to this end they must be sitting up during the entire time when they are giving the breast lest they fall asleep unawares while the child is nursing and smother it, having failed to take this necessary precaution.

Until the end of the seventeenth century the semiaccidental smothering of nurselings was tolerated as a "morally neutral fact, condemned by the ethics of Church and State, but practiced in secret, half-consciously and at the borderline of intention, forgetfulness, and clumsiness."[21] By the eighteenth century the family tended to value the child; but a new type of rejection manifested itself in the form of abandonment. Exposure of infants within two or three days of birth became increasingly prevalent, reaching massive proportions during the Revolution. A surge of tenderness and concern about the hereafter contributed to the decision to let the bastard child or the extra mouth live after all. As for the systematic "putting out to nurse" of the children of certain milieux (shopkeepers, artisans, the liberal professions), sometimes on the very day of their birth,[22] it amounts to a temporary rejection of the child and a form of indifference on the mother's part. These facts are well known and I simply evoke them here. I will add, however, that the immediate separation of mother from child and its speedy wrapping in constraining swaddling clothes are a legacy of Western civilization. As soon as the birth is over, there is no longer any physical intimacy between the mother and the child, no moment of tender love and fondling. The break is abrupt, as if it were a matter of erasing, as quickly as possible, the carnal reality of the child's life in the womb, that lost paradise. Beginning only some hours later, breast-feeding, if indeed it takes place, represents another form of special relationship.

The child to be born was a stranger. Its person assumed a place in the family only when it proved robust enough to have a chance of living. Yet, with the decline of infanticide, one notices different collective attitudes, tending toward respect for life and meticulous concern for survival. The many pleas for breast-feeding by the mother and against swaddling are classic examples. Surgeons sometimes charged midwives with responsibility for many infant deaths, dwelling at length on their own efforts at resuscitation when finding an inanimate newborn (mouth-to-mouth breathing, rubbing, shaking, applying packs, inserting a feather into the esophagus).[23] This did not happen often, for infant mortality hardly declined at all. One also wonders about the future mental capacity of children who were subjected to these efforts at resuscitation, sometimes for an hour or more. None of the eighteenth-century treatises addresses one fundamental question, namely, whether protracted labor and the strenuous efforts to "recover" the life of a stillborn child would result in a mass of defective or malformed children.

Concern for the new being is most evident in the obsession with baptism: no soul must be given over to damnation because it has not received baptism. In this connection the problem of fixing the moment when a life recognized by God has begun in the mother's womb was as pressing to the clergy of the past as it is to today's physicians, moralists, and legislators dealing with the matter of abortion. In the face of this insoluble problem, the theologians came to the conclusion that the child is entitled to baptism as soon as any part of its body, no matter which one, has emerged. In 1770 the instructions published by Michel Raulin at the behest of the government dwelt at extraordinary length on the religious duties of the midwife, the spiritual salvation of the mother, and the child's baptism.[24] These instructions contained a series of very strict formulations. The words of the baptism were to be preceeded by the words: "If you are human," "if you are capable of receiving baptism," or "if you are not baptized," as the case may be (misshapen child, inert child, impossible delivery). When the child was definitively trapped, the Church also recognized the validity of baptism by injection. At the end of the seventeenth century, especially in the climate created by the Revocation of the Edict of Nantes in Languedoc, the records of episcopal visitation indicate a new interest in the woman who practices midwifery in the parish. Is she capable? the questionnaires wanted to know. Capable of administering baptism, that is. "A time was to come, in the eighteenth century, when the midwife, that white witch, retrieved by the powers that be, was to be given the mission of protecting the child."[25] What is meant here is protection from heresy. As late as the eighteenth century, Protestant midwives did their work in secrecy, so as not to have to take the child to the church. Traces of legal proceedings have survived. In 1748 Anne Galinier was condemned for assisting a woman living by herself in her confinement and failing to have the child baptized. She was imprisoned for life despite her advanced age. She was almost eighty years old.[26]

Table 7.1 shows age at baptism in the parish of Saint-Fulcran at Lodève. For the seventeenth century, samples are taken from all years for which registers are available; for the eighteenth century, samples are taken at ten-year intervals.[27] Also in that period of the 1740s the Catholic authorities insisted that the child be baptized at home whenever it was in the slightest jeopardy, so the parish priest frequently went to private homes when it became clear that a difficult birth was ahead. This was the time when the Tridentine rule of baptism within three days was really followed, even though it had been largely disregarded in the preceeding two hundred years.

This haste to ensure the newborn's spiritual salvation intensified the existing anxiety and fear of the unknown; to some extent it also took matters out of the parents' hands. The mother's certainty that she was bringing forth an impure being, tainted by original sin, became one with the idea of defilement attached to the act of giving birth. Georges Witowski gives many examples of this feeling of shame, which is related to the shedding of blood and the ideal of virginity. Women retire, hide, and cover themselves.[28] In the most diverse civilizations, an endless number of rites of purification can be found (in Thai

Table 7.1 — Ages at Baptism As Listed in Saint-Fulcran Parish, Lodève

Year								Days									
	0	1	2	3	4	5	6	7	8	9	10	11	12	13	14	15	16 and +
1607			2	4	1	3	4	2	*8*		3	4	1	1	2	3	8
1642	2		2	1	1	7	3	3	8	5	5	2	4	3	2	1	30
1670	2	3	4	11	12	*21*	10	*21*	18	9	6	2		2	1	5	4
1680		6	*9*	9	4	2	1	1									
1695	2	15	28	*41*	27	30	22	11									
1705	0	17	32	27	*38*	37	34	24	6	2	1						
1715	3	16	20	27	*37*	27	27	32	9	1	1						
1725	7	34	47	*71*	42	10	3	7	1		1	1					
1738	28	61	*71*	49	20	2		1						1			
1745	24	*68*	63	36	16	2											1
1755	39	*85*	53	27	5						1						
1765	59	*103*	70	30	11	3	1										
1775	70	*94*	48	18	8	1	1										
1785	92	*124*	65	14	4												

Note: The totals do not represent the number of births but the number of baptisms for which the date of birth is indicated. The italicized figure represents the maximum, that is, the highest incidence of baptism at a given age.

The sampling for the seventeenth century is irregular due to gaps in the registers; sampling is at ten-year intervals for the eighteenth century.

society, all the windows are opened and the woman turns toward the east; Moslem women loosen their hair).[29] Ceremonies of "churching," which centered on the idea of purification, have now fallen into disuse, but our grandmothers still experienced them. Even now women are obviously held in thrall by this mental heritage; the feeling of shame, the idea of impurity, the passivity of the mother, all proceed from a cultural oppression that still exerts a tight hold over the women of our generation.

Pain and Violence

In past centuries, the pain of childbirth was always discussed in terms of a given, as a phenomenon that simply had to be endured. In the light of recent studies on the psychological control of pain, it may be possible to understand the suffering of women in childbirth as the weight of a thousand-year-old legacy constituted by such factors as feelings of impurity, frequently dramatic language and vocabulary, and the sense of guilt of the mother herself. Is it far-fetched to speak of a "pain complex of the Western world" and to see it expressed in seventeenth- and eighteenth-century France? "The traditional mode of childbirth in Western countries is indeed a cultural phenomenon, centered upon a preoccupation with pain and expressed through pain. At the same time, its fundamental reference point is the passivity with which women were made to submit."[30] Physicians of the eighteenth century touched very lightly on a problem that made them feel totally powerless. Questions about the nature of uterine contractions—the setting in motion and the mechanism of labor pains— were sometimes asked, but answers were never forthcoming. The physicians' resignation took the form of a minute description of the period of labor, from the "butterflies," the intermittent pains of the first hours, to the contractions of the stage of expulsion.

Throughout these accounts, the woman appears traumatized by previous confinements or by the many stories she has heard. The frequent occurrence of false labor, in which the woman convinced herself that the birth had begun, sometimes made for a labor of six or seven days. Were such cases due to erroneous perception on the part of the mother or to an anomalous labor that was constantly interrupted? However that may be, the time spent in labor was considerable (between twelve hours and three days), a fact that lent fuel to the legend of a heroic act. The woman gave violent expression to her pain: screaming, vomiting, convulsions, and fainting were commented upon by a female entourage that bemoaned her state and enacted a ceremonial of pain. To be sure, the accounts that have come down to us concern the most difficult births. They do not constitute a general mode. Yet they provoked and sustained a feeling of apprehension and tenseness that many generations were unable to overcome. The women who just dropped their children (*les perdeuses d'enfants*) and brought their babies home from the fields in their apron, and the pregnant girls who went off by themselves for an hour or so to give birth and then do away with their newborn, did not speak often and certainly did not write. They did little to attentuate an ancestral dread.

Ever since the publication of Dr. Engelmann's theories,[31] there has been widespread acceptance of the idea that the length of labor and the intensity of the pain felt increases with the degree of civilization. Engelmann was able to observe at first hand that among the tribes of Africa, Southern India, and Australia, births rarely take more than two hours. Rousseau's readers would not have disagreed with this idea. The labor of childbirth is probably easier for people living in a state of nature; such women, from mother to daughter, are less primed for suffering. But the ethnologists, even in the most recent studies, have more to say about feelings than about systematic observation.[32] Pain cannot be measured by the expression it is given. Some of the most primitive tribes do not permit any manifestation of pain, so that the stoic attitude of the women covers any emotion or despair. In Western society, the powerful conditioning for pain finds its expression and its justification in Christianity. The biblical curse is understood as divine vengeance and experienced as a sacrifice and an act of atonement. This attitude is as deeply rooted among the suffering poor as among the learned: "The female has been condemned by the author of nature to bring forth in pain. The labor of childbirth begins and ends with pain."[33] Here is a condemnation emanating from the depth of time, an impenetrable and terrifying precept that throughout the ages has stymied research, curiosity, and inventiveness, thus immobilizing childbirth in a ritual of suffering and violence.

Accusations of brutality and barbarity were bandied back and forth between the surgeons and the midwives of the "grand siècle," although their basic disagreement remains to be spelled out.[34] Can we go so far as to say that the woman in childbirth encountered "many forms of open or furtive sadism?"[35] Suffering certainly ceased to be a consideration when it came to separating the child from the mother as quickly as possible and at any cost; we hear of the irreversible prolapse of the uterus, tearing of the womb, rupturing of the "wall between the vulva and the anus which is vulgarly called the fork," brutal pulling out of the placenta, whole or in pieces,[36] and fatal hemorrhages. There was a collective awareness of the brutality endured by the mother, but this awareness was much more diffuse with respect to the child. Its birth was seen as a necessary ordeal not subject to questioning. If the child screamed and choked, it was a comforting sign that it was alive. It was shaken, beaten, imprisoned. If it was strong, it would live and assert itself.

For the people of that time, the horror of being born was found in more extreme situations, when children were condemned because the birth was mechanically impossible. In the books they wrote, the obstetricians never dared state the problem of choosing between the mother's and the child's life in forthright terms. Yet this problem arose every day when the child proved too large to pass through the pelvic passage once the head was engaged; since it was virtually impossible to perform an operation,[37] the desperate solution was to deliver the baby in pieces. There was no possibility of avoiding this practice once one had given up all hope in the natural process, the effect of medication, or the use of instruments. In 1782 one contemporary wit, most probably a surgeon of Montpellier, wrote a scathing pamphlet to be sent to the Estates of Languedoc, entitling it, "Petition by the Unborn Presented to the Gentlemen of the Estates of Languedoc in Connection with Their Charges against the So-Called Wise Women."* This is the only example of a document that has the fetus speak and express its terror of the adult world.

The charges concern, first of all, the fact that it is not safe for us to enter into this world. We dare show ourselves there only in fear and trembling, since we are continually mistreated by certain women they call matrons, who make bold to insult us in our cubicles, despite our care in keeping our doors closed. If we become annoyed, they lampoon and shame us, calling us rogues, rebels, and bandits. They bruise us, they skin us, they tear us to pieces without pity, and often treat us even worse than that. . . .[38]

This general acquiescence in brutality and fatalism did not exclude a willingness to help. But what could chivalrous declarations accomplish? "Since the amiable sex suffers the pains of childbirth only because it has shared man's pleasure, it is certainly right for us to do what we can to alleviate its suffering."[39] The women present at the delivery supported the woman in labor by the lower back while she was stretched out, and by the shoulders at the stage of expulsion. Whenever an obstetrician wrote about his experience, he devoted long passages to the posture the woman in childbirth was made to assume, and we learn that special chairs and short beds especially made for the purpose were gradually abandoned during the eighteenth century. The woman was placed at the edge of her own bed. "Two persons will be stationed at the foot of the bed in order to hold down her bent knees and prevent her from stretching her legs when the pains come. Two other persons, stationed at the head of the bed, will hold the patient's hands, which they will press when there is pain."[40]

In making a comparative inventory of the positions for delivery among all races, Dr. Engelmann doubted that the prone position adopted in France is the least difficult.[41] Could it be that it befits a mental attitude that sees the woman in childbirth as a sick person and a martyr? The great obstetricians of the eighteenth century, and some modest surgeons as well, were well aware that calm and confidence were more important than the posture of the woman in childbirth. Called very late to a delivery, with the woman exhausted and terrified, the obstetrician always made it his first business to reassure everyone involved, and sometimes this was sufficient to bring about a safe delivery. He knew by intuition and by experience that panic and tenseness intensify "the irritation and compression of the nerves that cause pain"[42] and that a cool head, patience, and assurance are more helpful to the mother than science. In 1786 Maître Rigal, a surgeon at the hospital of Gaillac near Albi and a correspondent of the Royal Academy of Montpellier, reported one of the miracles due to nothing more than his presence.

*This is a pun on the literal meaning of the term *sage-femme*—midwife.—Trans.

On the third day, when her strength was almost exhausted and her hopes were completely dashed—this was a young patient—it was decided to call on me for help. I found the patient with the pallor of despair upon her brow and her family in the most vivid distress. I immediately proceeded to a palpation in order to be fully informed of the situation. I found the labia majora bruised and inflamed as a result of manipulations that were as heavyhanded as they were misguided. I cautiously inserted my finger as far as the womb. I found its opening dilated to the size of a small coin. The child presented the top of its head, and since the necessary conditions for a normal birth were present, it seemed to me that the delivery would take place as soon as there were pains sustained by sufficient strength. In this manner I found that, despite the alarm spread by the inadequacy of the midwife, the situation was bad only to the extent that she had caused it to be so. I therefore concentrated all my efforts upon comforting the patient by assuring her that she would be safely delivered before long.[43]

But the practitioners of the eighteenth century did not carry their efforts to develop soothing language and manipulations very far. Their attitude was centered on providing relief and waiting. In a chapter on symbolic effectiveness, Claude Lévi-Strauss cites a long shamanic incantation used in a tribe of Cuna Indians (Panama) to speed up a delivery.[44] Even before psychoanalytic analysis became widely known, Lévi-Strauss showed that the woman in childbirth must be helped to become conscious of her conflicts and her resistance. In a civilization—that of the old France—where suffering and resignation were glorified, an emphasis on relief was out of place and pain continued to confer status.

For that same society birth and death existed side by side and became one and the same. The mortality of women in childbirth and of infants is no myth. To become aware of their reality, one can read through the memoirs of the obstetricians and the list of baptisms and deaths in the parish registers. In the annex volume to his treatise, François Mauriceau published an account of the 600 pathological cases in which he had intervened. On the basis of these memoirs one can establish a typology of the accidents of pregnancy and childbirth in the seventeenth century. It testifies to an objective reason for the fear of suffering and dying. (Cf. table 7.2.)

Of the 594 cases in this tragic inventory, 78 resulted in the death of the mother and 230 in that of the child. These figures cannot be translated into the real percentages of difficult births since they do not concern normal deliveries. While the enumeration of these cases provides some important indications, it would be unwise to place too much trust in these accounts, which may have been written long after the fact.

These accounts confirm the most dreaded anomalies encountered in childbirth, including inadequate dilation, which makes the child's passage physically impossible and dooms both the mother and the fetus; hemorrhaging at the time of the delivery; the cancerous ulcer, which progresses rapidly after the birth; death of the fetus in the womb; and finally the various postpartum fevers that were the object of ancestral dread. In the list of causes of death compiled from Mauriceau's memoirs, maternal mortality after an abortion or due to a fever is low; it must be kept in mind, however, that these are the

Table 7.2—Cases of Difficult Deliveries Cited by Mauriceau (March 1669-October 1693)

Symptom	Number of Cases	Mother Dies	Child Dies
Abortion	80	4	80
Labor of 5 to 8 days	6	3	3
Venereal disease	9	—	—
Consumption	2	2	—
Inflammation of the womb (attempted abortion)	12	3	—
Inversion of the womb	2	—	—
Premature breaking of the water	9	—	3
Ignored pregnancy	7	—	—
False pregnancy	1	—	—
Delirium, hysteria	7	2	1
Placenta born before child	4	2	1
Arm out up to shoulder	18	—	5
Foot and knee out	10	—	4
Facial presentation	7	—	3
Breech presentation	11	—	5
Cord hanging out	26	—	7
Cord knotted	7	—	—
Fetus not viable	26	—	—
Ulcer	35	16	1
Prolapse of the womb	—	—	—
Ten-month pregnancy	3	—	—
Vomiting	3	1	—
Convulsions	31	8	12
Rupture of the womb	2	—	1
Vulva torn to anus	2	—	1
Involuntary urination	3	—	—
Dysentery	5	3	4
Fever	30	7	4
Total or partial retention of placenta	25	2	1
Violence of midwives or surgeons	7	2	7
Dilation without delivery	5	5	5
Head wedged	7	—	6
Child too large	6	2	2
Deformed child	6	—	2
Child dead and putrefied	38	2	38
Twins	38	—	9
Triplets	1	—	1
Simulation of dropsy	4	—	—
Caesarian section on dead woman	3	3	—
Hemorrhage	94	11	21

Source: François Mauriceau, *Traité des maladies des femmes grosses et de celles qui sont accouchées* (Paris, 1792)

Note: In each of these cases, Mauriceau mentioned only the most outstanding symptom.

observations of a practicing obstetrician who saw his patient only for a few days, rather than a few weeks, after the delivery. But the terrifying impression left by these violent fits of fever marked the consciousness of the people and fueled a climate of terror. Some physicians have given us descriptions of these fevers or noted their numerical incidence in the hospitals. In the most serious cases, those that involved septicemia, the outward symptoms were shaking, anxiety, sunken eyes, severe abdominal pains, nausea, and delirium.[45] Owing to the mother's weakened defenses, the germs of infection were able to enter through the placental wound, some of these germs being autogenous (pieces of the membrane or the placenta, the dead fetus), others coming from the environment (unasepticized instruments, wound or fever of a contact person).

In the hospital milieu, puerperal infections remained quite prevalent until the era of systematic disinfection. For Nantes, René Baudard considers the 1880s decisive (between 1858 and 1869, childbed mortality due to fever at the Nantes hospital was 9.3 percent, a figure that fell to 1.1 percent after 1882).[46] This scourge affected above all the women who gave birth at the hospital—that is, the poor—where mortality was extemely high. François Doublet mentioned 12 cases of fever for the 60 women who had given birth in 1791 at the hospital of Vaugirard; in 1800 J. Baptiste Demangeon held the negligence of the personnel of the Hôtel-Dieu of Paris responsible for the fact that this institution had the highest mortality rate during and after delivery, namely, 1 in 10.[47] In the Berlin hospitals, 1 in 18 died, in those of Dublin 1 in 110, and in those of London 1 in 131. It is impossible to verify these figures. Nonetheless, they tell us something about the extraordinary carelessness with which childbirths were handled in French hospitals, where microbes were permitted to multiply freely and where the newly confined women were not isolated from the other patients. Paradoxically, those who were confined at home were less threatened.

By checking these indications against a detailed list of women deceased within the period of the confinement in the parish registers, one realizes that the mother's death dates are distributed over the entire month following the confinement. As a reference and as an example, I shall cite here the information about the women who died in childbirth or shortly thereafter found in one rural parish, Villeneuve-lès-Maguelonne, at the end of the seventeenth and in the eighteenth century (table 7.3).

A modest martyrology of women who died in childbirth, this list of some forty records isolated from the registers of a small town (600 inhabitants) in Languedoc over the span of a century (1681-1791) testifies to the numerical reality of the phenomenon. In this parish, where twenty to twenty-five children were born every year, approximately and on the average less than one woman died clearly in childbirth or shortly thereafter in any given two-year period. It is obvious that the parish registers are insufficient to establish a reliable list of all the cases of childbirth resulting in the mother's death. Children who died unbaptized, particularly premature ones, were rarely registered, especially before 1720; and for the period covering the reign of Louis XIV the attempt to find the women who died in childbirth yields even more disappointing results. Nonetheless, this series, small and in need of comparison with others as it is, opens up certain methodological perspectives and permits us to outline certain methodological questions.

At what age did women die in childbirth? Young wives (twenty-five to twenty-nine years) who were giving birth to their first or second child died as often as overburdened mothers (forty to forty-four years). When did death occur in relation to the delivery? On the same day, of course, or, more

Table 7.3—Childbed Mortality at Maguelonne at the End of the Seventeenth Century and in the Eighteenth Century

The Mother			The Confinement				The Family		
Name	Age	Date	Days Elapsed Between Confinement and Death	Sex of Child	Child in Danger	Years of Marriage	Total Number of Children	Children Died Young
Marguerite Barelle, wife of Jean Cayzergues, shepherd	25	July 1689	31	M	—	1	1	—
Catherine Viguiere, wife of François Canebié, plowman	40	June 1699	7	F	—	4	2	—
Marie Darles, wife of St. Etienne Donnadieu	34	Sept. 1701	20	M	—	—	8	3
Elisabeth Bouladonne, wife of Antoine Boudon, plowman	35	Oct. 1706	25	F	—	11	5	
Antoinette Laurence, wife of Pierre Boudon, worker	35	Sept. 1711	10	M	died at 10 days	—	4	1
Suzanne Libourel, wife of Etienne Bouladou, plowman	27	March 1718	12	M	—	6	3	
Catherine Saunier, wife of noble Jean Astruc, king's councilor	20	Dec. 1724	0	F	—	—	—	—
Suzanne Melgue, wife of Daniel Bourrely	40	Jan. 1727	30	M	baptized	—	—	—
Suzanne Peyre, wife of Pierre Olivier	27	April 1730	32	F	—	2	1	—
Marie-Anne Couston, wife of Antoine Suquet	25	Dec. 1731	31	F	—	5	3	—
Marguerite Donnat, wife of Eulorand Barral	25	March 1734	0	F	baptized, buried	3	2	—

Jean Pinquier, surgeon

Name	Age	Date		Sex				
Jeanne Lacroix, wife of Etienne Peire, worker	30	July 1736	31	F	—	12	4	—
Anne Donnadieu, wife of St. Jean Goudard, bourgeois, *viguier*	41	Nov. 1736	0	F	—	15	9	4
Marie Soulié, wife of Raimond Salva, worker	28	Jan. 1737	21	M	—	5	2	—
Marie Ebrard, wife of St. Louis Bouislet, shopkeeper	—	Jan. 1740	0	F	—	—	—	—
Marguerite Cambié, wife of Jean Crespin, cottager	24	June 1740	6	F	died at 12 days	1	1	1
Catherine Desaudrieux, wife of Sr. Louis Paul, captain coast guard	27	Sept. 1741	0	M	—	5	4	1
Marie Guilhard, wife of St-Antoine Crespin	35	Feb. 1744	0	F	died at 3 weeks	10	4	3
Marie Rouanet, wife of Pierre Uziol, worker	35	Nov. 1747	29	M	—	7	3	2
Jeanne Piquier, wife of Jean Plazen, worker	27	1747	5	M	baptized	2	1	—
Brigitte Cambié, wife of Antoine Ratier, worker	38	May 1749	6	M	—	19	7	—
Catherine Verdier, wife of Antoine Delor, worker	36	Oct. 1750	4	F	baptized	6	3	—
Catherine Martin, wife of Vital Co heiri,	40	Dec. 1751	9	FF	twins baptized	1	2	—

Table 7.3 (continued)

The Mother			The Confinement			The Family		
Name	Age	Date	Days Elapsed Between Confinement and Death	Sex of Child	Child in Danger	Years of Marriage	Total Number of Children	Children Died Young
worker								
Marie Grollier, wife of Benoît Verdier, cottager	36	Oct. 1759	15	F	died at 1 day	—	—	—
Catherine Tiei, wife of Jean Cuminal, worker	36	Nov. 1759	11	F	—	—	—	—
Marque Dorue, wife of Pierre Gervais	30	March 1763	35	F	—	13	6	3
Marianne Prinquier, wife of Pierre Viguier, cottager	25	March 1764	13	M	—	—	—	—
Elisabeth Fourquier, wife of Etienne Valette, fisherman	33	Dec. 1770	5	M	baptized	11	5	1
Thérèse Peire, wife of Pierre Boudon, cottager	40	Feb. 1776	10	M	—	18	7	3
Louise Puech, wife of Guillaume Roustan	30	Oct. 1780	7	M	—	7	4	2
Catherine Lauzet, wife of Jean Dufat	28	Feb. 1782	27	F	—	4	2	1
Jeanne Tinel, wife of Jean Vassas, cottager	44	May 1782	4	F	—	24	9	3
Anne Coulon, wife of Jacques Jac,	26	July 1785	3	M	—	3	2	—

of Antoine Bourdol								
Jeanne Lauzet, wife of Etienne Bourde, fisherman	27	Sept. 1787	3	M	died soon	—	—	—
Catherine Chauvet, wife of Jean Chauvet, fisherman	26	May 1788	18	M	—	5	3	1
Marguerite Veissière, wife of Mathieu Berganion, fisherman	25	April 1970	26	M	—	—	—	—
Marie Ramadier, wife of Pierre Bir, cottager	30	June 1791	17	F	—	—	—	—

frequently, considerably later (either within the first ten days or around the thirtieth day). On the basis of these indications—which must, of course, be confirmed by the study of longer series—it is possible to formulate some hypotheses concerning the pathological process leading to death. It would seem that the cases of quick death corresponded to a hemorrhage. Death was immediate whenever the woman was badly torn, that is, if the placenta or the child were pulled out too violently, and in such cases the child as well frequently died. In other cases the mother would gradually die of irremediable loss of blood within three or four days. When the mother died between the sixth and the thirtieth cays—and it is impossible to set a strict time limit—she usually succumbed to a more or less rapidly evolving puerperal fever.

The example of Villeneuve-lès-Maguelonne seems to suggest that until the end of the eighteenth century puerperal fever remained the dominant cause of death in childbirth. We find many cases of immediate death until about 1730; subsequently there were fewer of these, which suggests that the medical profession was beginning to deal more effectively with the mechanical aspects of birth, but not with infection. Finally, one wonders whether in this village the wives of notables were better protected than the others. It appears that until 1750 this was not the case. For the first period this list of burials shows as many wives of plowmen, bourgeois, merchants, officeholders, and even nobles as wives of small artisans and day laborers. By contrast, in the 1760s, '70s, and '80s, all the women who died following a delivery were wives of workers, cottagers (ménagers), or fishermen. The rich and respectable classes lived in better hygienic conditions, tended to restrict the number of children they had, and shunned the services of midwives, calling instead upon the more competent surgeons. At that point, the death of a woman in childbirth was usually related to poverty and ignorance.

In preindustrial societies, the birth of a child did indeed constitute a risk and a source of anxiety, as the study of these quantitative series very clearly shows. In addition, however, the revolting aspect of the death of a woman at the time when she gave birth to a child could only exacerbate the feeling of fear and defenselessness in the collective imagination. The statistical correlation between the women who died during their childbearing years (age nineteen to forty-five) and those who are positively known to have died in childbirth yields a low figure. Between 1686 and 1789 at Villeneuve-lès-Maguelonne it was 40 in 284, or 1 in 7. Moreover, the comparison of death figures for men and women between the ages of nineteen and forty-five yields very conflicting results, suggesting that women of childbearing age were not decimated. A sampling shows that at Clermont-l'Hérault 38 women and 17 men in that age bracket died between 1698 and 1700; between 1750 and 1752 the figure was 34 women and 30 men. At Maugio the same sample yields the figures 8 and 10 for the period 1698-1700 and 4 and 11 for the period 1750-52; and in Saint Ann's parish at Montpellier the figures were 51 and 42 in 1698-1700 and 39 and 38 in 1750-52.[48]

Men died at the same rate, almost, from accidents or epidemics. Dying in the aftermath of giving birth remained an individual tragedy. Yet the fright of the mothers passed down through the generations, and their ignorance and their psychological conditioning, together with the legend of the midwife, made it into a collective tragedy.

Who Were the Incompetent Matrons?

Whenever a confinement took place, the women of the family or the neighborhood seemed to fulfill a social function. The exclusion of the male is a general pattern. Comparing the behavior and the attitudes of primitive peoples in North and South America, North Africa, Black Africa, and Southeast Asia, Bernadette Bonnet notes that almost everywhere the child's father and all male occupants must leave the house, to be replaced by some female relatives and neighbors who come to attend the mother. The husband is called only if something goes wrong with the confinement.[49] Very much the same attitude prevailed in the families of old France. To what extent have today's women in childbirth overcome this age-old desire? Do they not in many cases prefer the attendance of a midwife to that of a physician, and the presence of their mother to that of their husband? The mere fact that deliveries in the family home have fallen out of favor and that births now take place in the unfamiliar surroundings of antiseptic hospital rooms does not testify to new patterns of behavior.

The fear of being indecent, the fear of being dishonored, the fear of being seen in the throes of suffering—these great ageless concerns were at the core of the debate over "the indecency of having men deliver women."[50] By the eighteenth century the surgeons, having formed an increasingly powerful guild, had acquired a certain competence in difficult cases and were often called to attend women in childbirth—reluctantly, yet with great faith. Philippe Hecquet advanced a number of arguments against their intervention, claiming that ancient history gives examples of learned midwives, that the tenets of Christian religion are incompatible with the profession of obstetrician, that women are as capable of conducting a delivery as men, and that the coquetry of young women can be boundless. Many published responses to this pamphlet simply considered it ridiculous.[51] And so it was; yet it testifies to a genuine uneasiness. Most of the treatises in defense of the surgeons used the argument that midwives were ignorant and reckless. By the end of the century, the debate broadened and the controversy spilled over into some highly significant areas.

The small book by Elisabeth Nihell published in 1771 in support of midwives[52] shows how easily a surgeon, called in at a critical moment, could gain ascendency over the woman in childbirth and her entire family. Her argumentation includes an analysis of the strategy of seduction. "To what dangers will not her virtue be exposed if she thinks herself pretty enough to deserve the attention of her obstetrician, at the very least a compliment from him on the secret charms he will have examined; all of which will flatter her all the more as it comes from a visitor who, given his many opportunities for comparison, is bound to be considered an expert in the matter by the pretty lady." Elisabeth Nihell intuitively understood the power wielded by an indispensible male, his role as father figure and sage. "She will be susceptible to the kind of weakness that makes her imagine that she is completely dependent on a man who wields great power over her as it is, seeing that he is her obstetrician, so that she will permit him to gain greater ascendency over her and her family than a midwife would ever think of." Elisabeth Nihell also criticized reckless operations performed without consulting the family. "When this tragic operation is finished, what is there to comfort you except perhaps the positive assertion on the part of the clever doctor that if such violence had not been used, the mother would have been lost along with the child."

When faced with this choice, the women—at least in urban areas—may well have followed a trend of fashion. Once the royal example had been set by Louis XIV, who called the obstetrician Julien Clément to Mademoiselle de La Vallière's childbed, the surgeons' guild began to gain recognition among ladies of quality and in very difficult cases. In the countryside, where the obstetrician was sometimes called from far away, he was only brought in at the last extremity, after three or four days of alleged labor. Powerless because he had come so late, or because his means for dealing with difficult cases were limited, he was always an outsider. In the village, the reign of the midwife continued.

The matron of old France was an imposing figure. Her age, her experience, or at least her familiarity with the course of a confinement, conferred authority upon her. She was called as soon as a woman felt, or believed she felt, the first pains. She knew the history of the family better than anyone. In the oaths taken by the midwives, one frequently finds the formula: "I promise not to divulge the secrets of families or persons I shall attend." She covered up any scandal connected with an illegitimate birth. She was expected to be helpful but discreet. If she reached old age, she had seen the birth of many of the village's or neighborhood's inhabitants. In the course of the eighteenth century, the role of the midwife gradually detached itself from the idea that it was a social function and became a profession. Some practiced for a month or two with a surgeon.[53] Some, who became famous for their skill, have left collections of advice. One of these was Louise Bourgeois, midwife to Marie de Medicis;[54] others were Marguerite de la Marche[55] and Anne-Marie Le Boursier Du Coudray.[56]

The last of these women assumed an educational task and had the idea of using mannequins to illustrate the theoretical courses she conducted in various provinces.[57] Her itinerant ministry was a gesture of revolt. A relatively isolated phenomenon, it did not have any immediate effect on the lack of knowledge and the fatalism prevailing at the time.[58]

The practice of midwifery only became a real profession recognized by certification with the laws of the Directory and the [Napoleonic] Empire, which called for obstetrical training centers in the chief town of each department.[59] Until that time, midwives had no status. One might wonder at the severity, indeed the acrimony, with which they were treated by surgeons and administrators, especially in rural areas. Our sources are obviously misleading; for testimonies of support and trust were not written down, while an entire polemical literature has come down to us. The struggle for influence, which in the eighteenth century erupted into a violent quarrel between surgeons and midwives, has left its mark on every treatise on childbirth. Among many examples, here is one passage from François Mauriceau's treatise:

There are certain midwives who are so afraid that the surgeon will take their practice away from them, or that they will appear ignorant in his presence, that they would rather take the greatest chances than send for the surgeon when it becomes necessary. Others are so presumptuous that they think they are as capable of undertaking everything as the surgeon. One also finds some who, from a lack of knowledge and experience in their art, keep hoping in vain that the child will eventually assume the right position, and that mishaps will right themselves (if it pleases God, as they say). Some intentionally arouse in the poor women such fear and apprehension of the surgeons, whom they describe as butchers and executioners, that the women sometimes would rather die in labor with the child in their belly than put themselves into the surgeon's hands.[60]

The second volume of the *Traité des femmes grosses et accouchées*, describing hundreds of desperate cases in which his intervention was necessary,[61] is a permanent indictment of the midwives' incompetence. But should we completely accept it? Philippe Peu makes no distinction between the foolish and pretentious midwife and the "throng of babbling females" surrounding the women in childbirth; he has a smile for superstitions and amulets. "It must be admitted that if the obstetrician ever has a light moment, amidst the groans and screams that constantly assail his ears, it comes on the occasions when the old-time crones unpack their fanciful ideas with a pretention and a stubbornness at which one is hard-put to keep from laughing, although one is often obliged (when it does not matter) to let them have their way without objecting."[62] Aside from "a heavy weight of rosaries and medals," the most prevalent practices for speeding up the birth of a child and ensuring its health included lighting a tall candle, soaking a rose of Jericho, and rubbing the mother's mouth with a gold coin. (This recalls the traditional midwife in Muslim coutries, who uses the tricks of the trade handed down by old matrons and is quick to forget what she may have learned in European hospitals. She is an elderly woman, incapable of absorbing new ideas. In difficult cases, her attitude is one of withdrawal and fatalism.)[63] One is struck to see that in pre-industrial or traditional societies the midwife represents respect for tradition, a ritualistic attitude and, by the same token, resistance to new ideas.

Michel Raulin, whose official study was published in 1770, does not qualify his accusations in any way. "Every day they cause both mother and child to perish, since they lack the knowledge necessary and required to save them. They often mutilate both mother and child to the point of weakening them for life and causing them to become a burden to themselves and useless to society."[64] Among all the indictments of the matrons who acted as midwives, the most virulent and courageous example, a most intriguing document for the historian of Languedoc, is still the "Petition of the Unborn," which I have cited above as an extravagant and eye-opening piece of raillery.

Nonetheless, it is clear that more and more frequently the midwives of the eighteenth century called in a surgeon when the birth proved to be "against nature." This obligation was included in most of the texts of their oath of office. Here one already sees the first manifestations of a subordination to the surgical profession that was to be a portent of things to come. Today's midwife very rarely performs beyond the limits of a normal birth. She is far from being accorded the respect enjoyed by the obstetrician. She turns the case over to him at the moment of the actual birth and whenever a complication arises. Yet if something goes wrong, the obstetrician and the woman's family consider it her fault.[65]

In the bundles of correspondence on the subject of midwives exchanged between the local authorities and the subdelegates (surveys of 1737 and 1786)[66] the dominating theme is, once again, the verdict of ignorance. The statements for each subdelegation submitted in response to the survey of 1786 constantly use such expressions as "the women deliver each other" (Le Vigan), "learned from her mother, does routine work, no regular practice" (Tournon), "the unfortunate victims are forced to submit to their ineptitude" (Le Puy), "50 matrons spread throughout these villages without the right to practice and without training, adhering to a blind and murderous routine" (Narbonne), "midwives from mother to daughter over four generations" (Anduze), "all they do is let nature take its course" (Agde). The midwives did not know how to read or write. The subdelegates' letters for Agde, Mende, and Barre expressly stated that it was impossible to submit a list of midwives. "The ineptitude of these women is so great that if the birth is not normal, mother and child will perish." Lost among a flood of complaints, occasional evidence that the villagers had confidence in the effectiveness of long experience comes to light. Such rare tributes were submerged in a rising tide of anger. One can more or less clearly follow the midwives of the various parishes through specific statements in the baptismal records, for these records note the occasions when a midwife privately baptized a child at home if she considered its life in danger, when she presented an illegitimate child to the priest, and when she served as witness or godmother, as she often did. These indications were given more or less consistently, depending on the period.

From some detailed remarks one gathers that a certain number of village women occasionally served as midwives. Their names appear only once or twice, and it is unlikely that they were approved by the bishop. By contrast, from the end of the seventeenth to the end of the eighteenth century, every given parish had two or three midwives who regularly delivered the local women for as long as thirty-five years. Sometimes one can even follow them from mother to daughter. At Maugio, fifteen midwives were named, each for very short periods of two to five years. Only one of them, whose name appears between 1703 and 1720, attended women in childbirth for almost twenty years. At Villeneuve-lès-Maguelonne during the same period, this function did not become a separate thing from lending a neighborly hand until 1750. Most of the women whose competence was sought were elderly housewives, often widows. They began practicing when their youngest child was grown up. (See table 7.4.)

Table 7.4—Midwives Cited in the Registers of Villeneuve-les-Maguelonne between 1698 and 1791

Year	Midwife
1693	Anne Domergue
1694	Suzanne Duboit
1698	Catherine Berenice
1700-1701	Antoinette Beysse
1701-9	Marie Malette
1708	Claire Bouladonne
1712-16	Anne Cayzergue
1720-30	No recorded home baptisms
1741	Marguerite Autié
1743	Marguerite Couston
1749-65	Magdeleine Salva
1768-77	Jeanne Fabre
1770-87	Anne Bringuière
1781	Jeanne Plazen
1782	Anne Vidale
1784	S. Glaize

Some of these cases are typical. Marguerite Autié served as midwife around 1741. Fifty-one years old, she was the wife of Jacques Bertrand, a fisherman by whom she had had nine children. Her youngest daughter was eight years old. Jeanne Fabre was the parish's midwife between 1768 and 1777. When she began to practice, she was fifty-five years old, and her children were between thirty and sixteen. A widow for the last eight years, she had been married to Jean Plazen, a rural laborer and farm hand at a large estate of Villeneuve. Invariably coming from very modest family backgrounds, the women who helped out other women were probably paid in kind, and stingily at that. There are no records of financial transactions between individuals, any more than there is a trace of wages paid by the community. But one does find many appeals to the bishop soliciting his approval of a midwife spontaneously chosen by the parishioners. Official requests by a municipal council asking a midwife to establish herself in the community and thereby offering her a quasi-public position are very rare. One example is furnished by Sète, perhaps because it was a town that had been very small in the past, because its demographic expansion was recent, and because the municipality had traditionally played a rather minor role. In 1756 a deliberation of the town council called for the installation of an experienced midwife:

The public complains that a town like ours, which is becoming more considerable each day, has only one midwife, who moreover is quite advanced in years, and that it frequently happens that several women are in labor at the same time, so that they must remain unattended, since that one woman cannot possibly deliver all of them. [It is therefore felt] to be in the public interest to find another midwife with good experience in this profession. Consequently, when widow Tarral of the village of Marseillan presented herself some time ago, offering to serve in this capacity, and when upon inquiry the council received a letter written on her behalf by the mayor and the consuls of Marseillan, stating that she is experienced in the conduct of a delivery, [it was decided that] steps should be taken to have her approved by Monseigneur the bishop of Agde as an indispensable necessity.[67]

Other sources that can be used are the various lists of midwives drawn up by the bishops, the intendants, and later the prefects. In 1684 and the following years, the parish censuses of the diocese of Montpellier (the questionnaires were prepared at the behest of Mgr. de Pradel and sent to the parish priests), indicate the presence of a midwife in a given community.[68] For the same diocese, the minutes of the first episcopal inspection tour of Mgr. Colbert (1698-99) mention the presence, name, marital status, training, and age of the midwife in each parish.[69] The surveys of 1737 and 1786, cited above, covered the entire intendancy of Languedoc. Finally, beginning with the [Napoleonic] Empire, the regulation of the profession provides a precise record of those who were inscribed on the official lists.[70] It is, therefore, possible to draw up comparative maps (see fig. 7.5). It is understood that such graphic representations cannot be altogether exact, for during the Ancien Régime neither the profession of obstetrician nor that of midwife was clearly defined. When it came to surgeons or barbers, women of experience or young trainees, their functions included border areas that were difficult to define in a survey. They were interpreted differently from region to region. In the two neighboring dioceses of Mirepoix and Limoux, the difference in the findings is extraordinary. At Mirepoix, the administrators included all the responses of the villages in which a woman practiced midwifery, listing 137 women, that is, almost 1 for each community, all of whom were between forty and fifty years old. At Limoux, 27 women were listed for 70 communities, all of them between twenty-five and thirty-five years old. (See figs. 7.6 and 7.7.) But here the administrators listed only those midwives who had taken the courses instituted in the last two years. The maps showing the distribution of midwives by diocese (fig. 7.7) thus provide certain indications but do not constitute reliable data. Table 7.5 shows the number of surgeons and midwives in the census of Languedoc of 1737.

Assuming that, generally speaking, the responses of the dioceses listed the number of women who systematically attended women in childbirth in their community—whether recognized by the ecclesiastical or medical authorities or not—the map based on the survey of Languedoc of 1737 suggests the

Table 7.5—Number of Surgeons and Midwives Reported for Languedoc in 1737

Diocese	Number of Communities Responding	Number of Surgeons	Number of Midwives
Agde	19	60	30
Alais	22	54	31
Albi	51	109	2
Alet	34	42	2
Béziers	69	102	84
Bas-Montauban	24	53	25
Carcassonne	26	59	27
Castres	31	60	27
Lavaur	23	61	16
Le Puy	25	38	9
Lodève	15	32	4
Mende	38	55	10
Mirepoix	40	42	21
Montpellier	47	109	54
Narbonne	49	89	2
Nimes	38	104	9
Rieux	38	47	46
St-Papoul	17	33	3
St-Pons	12	32	8
Toulouse	68	155	111
Uzès	59	109	22
Viviers	68	102	44

following hypotheses: the number of expert women was higher in dioceses that included a major urban center; and the women in such a diocese not only had the opportunity of practicing for a few years with a surgeon or in a hospice, but their slightly higher level of literacy was also more likely to place them into a position of responsibility. (Toulouse, Béziers, and Montpellier are illustrations of this situation.) By contrast, the outlying dioceses in relation to the main cities counted very few midwives (Albi, Alet, and Limoux). In the dioceses of Mende and Le Puy, this isolation from the cultural centers was even more pronounced in the mountainous areas. In very large dioceses, the number of midwives was extremely small. From this one should not conclude that, on the one hand, plain spells knowledge, and, on the other, mountain spells lack of culture.[71] Rather, one should realize that new regulations could be brought more easily to the lowlands of Languedoc, so that there the task of the midwife was more rapidly specified in the law. In marginal areas, this task was still largely a matter of mutual help.

The map of surgeons, also drawn up for 1737, contains similar information. The many surgeons of the lowlands, practicing close to the schools where they had been trained, aspired to medical status. In the mountains, they were much more dispersed; they were barbers rather than surgeons, and they rarely made house calls for a confinement. At that date, the census figures for

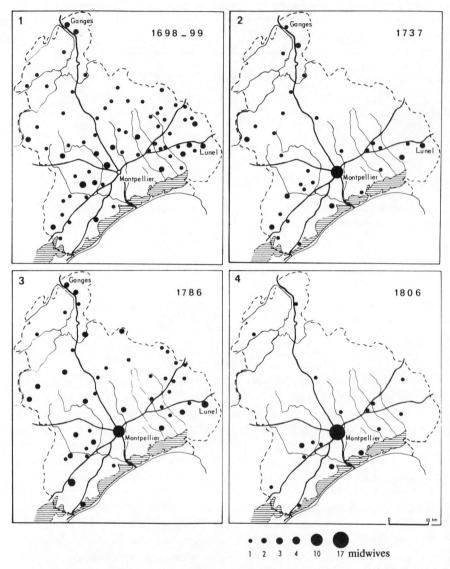

•	•	•	●	⬤	⬤
1	2	3	4	10	17 midwives

1. According to the pastoral visitations of Mgr. Colbert
2. According to the survey of 1737
3. According to the survey of 1786
4. According to the list of midwives practicing in the department of Hérault in 1806

Figure 7.5. Midwives in the Diocese of Montpellier

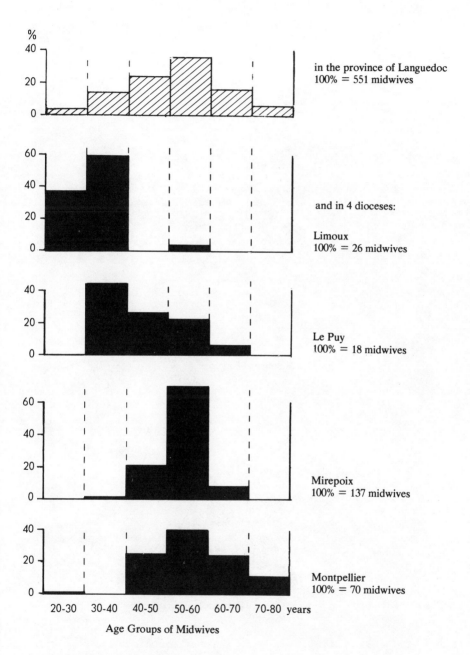

Figure 7.6. Distribution of Midwives by Age Groups (Percentages), According to the Survey of 1786

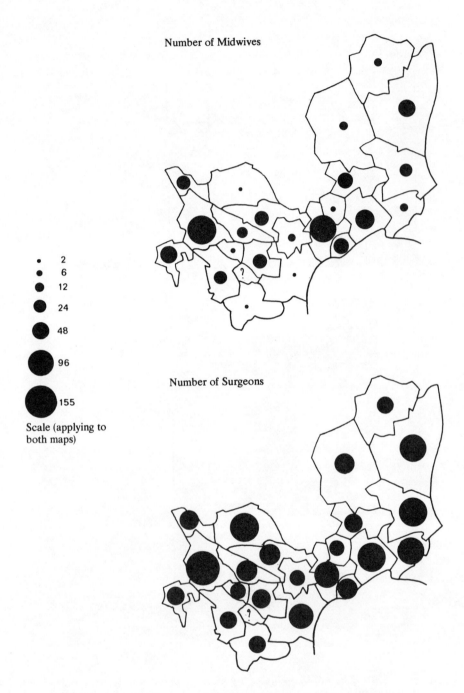

Figure 7.7. Number of Midwives and Number of Surgeons in Languedoc

surgeons were everywhere roughly twice those for midwives. The comparative maps showing the censuses of midwives in the diocese of Montpellier corroborate the slow emergence of professional status. Between 1698 (minutes of the episcopal visitation of Mgr. Colbert) and 1806 (licenses granted by the prefect's office, counted within the limits of the former diocese), the number of women practicing midwifery declined from 99 to 21 in an area comprising some 100 communities. They practiced, respectively, in 73 and 18 communities, excepting Montpellier (where figures for 1689 are not available). In 1732, 47 midwives were counted in 34 parishes; in 1786, there were 68 for 46 communities. In the middle of the eighteenth century, before the major regulations were instituted, the number of competent women increased. A profile of these women by marital status and age provides an even better definition of the typical matron practicing midwifery in the Languedoc of the 1780s. The person we find in parish after parish is a widow in half of the cases, fifty-one years old on the average (with a heavy cluster in the vicinity of forty-seven or forty-eight years, and again at fifty-two years). One wonders whether these women were of any real service beyond the age of sixty and until eighty (139 were in that age bracket in Languedoc in 1786). On the other hand, at the end of the eighteenth century, one finds the first examples of young midwives in their thirties, a phenomenon unknown in the seventeenth century. This is one more proof that competence and physical strength were beginning to supersede respect for age in people's minds (see fig. 7.8).

To Intervene or to Let Nature Take Its Course: An Unresolved Debate

In the field of obstetrics, as in all others, the men of the eighteenth century mounted a campaign against ignorance involving efforts at explanation and dissemination of information and a determination to defend their theories and ideas. Beginning with the 1680s, we find a profusion of pamphlets. Every author justified his undertaking in the preface by citing the pressing need for knowledgeable midwives. Pretentions ranged from the small pamphlet to the heavy treatise (Baudeloque's work of 1796 had 1,000 pages). The tone of these works is always deliberately pedagogical, to the point that some proceed by questions and answers. The title, *Catechisme de l'art d'accoucher* [Catechism of the art of midwifery], to which I have already alluded several times, is most suggestive in its wording. These works were probably learned by heart. They were scantily illustrated, if at all, sometimes showing a few anatomical sketches. The most heavily illustrated instructions are those of Marguerite de la Marche, who published plates showing dissections performed at the Hôtel-Dieu as early as 1710. The organization of these works was always essentially the same: pregnancy, description of labor and delivery, advice to watch the mother very carefully (it was recognized that the danger and the need for vigilance were greatest in the first hours after the delivery), advice for the care

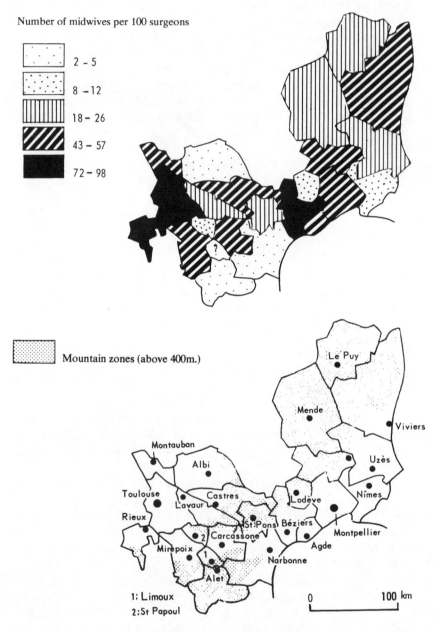

Number of midwives per 100 surgeons

2 – 5
8 – 12
18 – 26
43 – 57
72 – 98

Mountain zones (above 400m.)

Le Puy

Mende

Viviers

Montauban

Albi

Uzès

Toulouse
Castres
Lodève
Nîmes

Lavaur

Rieux

St Pons
Béziers

Montpellier

Carcassone
Agde

Mirepoix

Narbonne

Alet

1: Limoux
2: St Papoul

0   100 km

Figure 7.8. Number of Midwives in Relation to the Number of Surgeons in the Dioceses of the Province of Languedoc

of the newborn infant, and, above all, a presentation of all the "unnatural" fetal positions that would make the birth difficult or impossible. Frequently a third of the booklet was devoted to those unfortunate positions in which a child is unable to emerge without help from the outside: 150 of the 400 pages in the work by Pierre Amand[72] and 40 of the 84 pages in that of P. Anger du Fot, one of the rare catechisms of midwifery to be published at Montpellier.[73] To an extent that is impossible to determine, "unnatural" fetal positions may have been more frequent in the past than they are today. Baudeloque's catechism devotes 125 pages to bad positions that call for manipulations: presentations of the face, front of the neck, chest, abdomen, pelvis and thighs, back of the head, nape of the neck, small of the back, side of the head, shoulder, hand, chest, hip, and so forth. One senses a disproportionate interest in mishaps, an obsession with impossible situations.

Actually, these publications served very little purpose, for there was only one method that could improve the performance of the illiterate midwives — practical teaching. The efforts in this direction of Anne-Marie Le Boursier du Coudray have already been cited. This lady understood that many midwives were incapable of benefiting from printed books since they sometimes did not know how to read. Called in by royal governors and intendants who were curious about and interested in her work, she set up courses in province after province. Her great invention was a mannequin representing the mother and the fetus that enabled her to demonstrate the various manipulations. Wherever possible, lower-class women about to give birth were brought in, so that the students could gain practical experience in a hospice. A timid beginning was made in practical teaching. Madame Le Boursier appeared in Auvergne and in Burgundy, at Moulins, Besançon, Limoges, La Rochelle, Auch, Montauban, Grenoble, Châlons, Verdun, Amiens, Lille, and Caen. In 1759 she was authorized to conduct public courses of instruction in all provinces of the kingdom by letters patent from the king. An anonymous and undated memorandum deposited at the Bibliothèque Nationale [Paris] claims that she taught 4,000 students over a period of ten years. Sometimes her arrival was preceded by the creation of an official teaching institution. Courses of midwifery were instituted at the principal colleges of surgery: at Strasbourg in 1728 and at Paris in 1745 at the initiative of La Peyronne. In 1770, Montpellier's School of Surgery received statutes establishing courses in midwifery for matrons or midwives who were at least twenty-seven years of age, Catholic, able to read and write, and had practiced for at least two years in a hopital, with a surgeon, or with a trained midwife. The training sessions, purely theoretical in nature, lasted an hour and a half.[74] The real originator of obstetrical teaching at Montpellier was Jean Sénaux. Following the establishment of the School of Midwifery at the most important hospital of the department under the law of 9 ventôse, year X [1802], Sénaux became professor of midwifery at Saint-Eloi hospital.[75]

The more widespread practice of providing training for midwives appears to have spawned both continuous technical progress and a new attitude, expressed in an eagerness to intervene in the delivery and in injudicious attempts to perform dangerous manipulations and operations. Surgeons and trained midwives were only too glad to demonstrate their mastery.

I asked to be taken to one of those midwives who take on students and receive young people seeking instruction in the field of midwifery. There I saw examples of an inhumanity that would be almost incredible among barbarians. These midwives, hoping to attract large numbers of spectators, that is, payers of admission, have their emissaries announce that they have a woman in labor whose child would surely be born unnaturally. People flock to the scene and, in order not to disappoint their expectation, they will turn the child in the womb, causing it to be born feet first.[76]

This is an extreme and inhuman case. Nonetheless it proves that some midwives had become highly skilled in manipulating the child and in acting like a surgeon. Some knew how to find and bring down the feet, how to change the position of the fetus by deftly inserting their finger into its mouth, and how to respect and encourage the child's rotation at the moment of birth. One of the most famous obstetrical procedures was Mauriceau's, which is still known today by this name:

There are children whose head is so large that it becomes wedged in the passage after the body is already completely delivered, despite all the precaution one may have taken to avoid this situation. In this case, there is no point in simply tugging at the child by its shoulders, for sometimes one could more easily tear it off at the neck than bring it out in this manner. Instead, while some other person lightly pulls the child's body, holding it by the feet or above the knees, the surgeon must gradually disengage the child's head from between the bones of the passage. This he will do by first gently inserting two or three fingers of his left hand into the child's mouth in order to free its chin as a first step, then he will cradle the back of the child's neck with his right hand and pull with the fingers of his left hand placed in the child's mouth as I have described in order to free the chin, for it is this part that contributes most to fixing the head in the passage, from which it cannot be pulled before the chin is entirely disengaged.[77]

Today obstetricians consider this maneuver archaic, citing the danger of asphyxiation, intercranial lesion, or fracture of the shoulder blade, but they still refer to Mauriceau.

Midwives seem to have been more reluctant than surgeons to use instruments, which terrified the young women and ruined their confidence. As a desperate last measure, they used hooks—which looked like medieval instruments of torture to the eighteenth-century person—if the child was dead in the mother's womb or if the passage was too narrow, and this amounted to the conscious sacrifice of the child. French physicians made improvements in the forceps, which had been in use in Holland and England since the seventeenth century.[78] I am not interested here in chronicling the technical progress of apparatuses and operations, but, rather, in showing that the improvement of the forceps and its widespread use gave the surgeons a chance of bringing a difficult delivery to a conclusion without mutilating or dismembering the child. While the use of the forceps did not rule out brutal or clumsy handling, it did become more widespread.

This was not true for the operations that might permit a miraculous birth when the child was too large or badly positioned. Symphysis of the pubic bone or Caesarean sections were acts of bravura. The barbaric side of these operations—the absence of anesthesia, and the tragic atmosphere in which they took place (several women of the neighborhood were called in to hold down the mother after several days of fruitless labor), the virtual certainty that the mother, and the child as well, would die—gave rise to passionate controversy. All the eighteenth-century manuals for use by midwives treat this subject with reserve. They cite François Rouffet, doctor of medicine of Montpellier, who in 1581 had published a "new treatise on hysterotomotoxia or Cesarian birth, which is the extraction of the child by lateral incision of the womb of the pregnant woman unable to give birth otherwise, and this without prejudice to the life of one or the other." The manuals also show that Ambroise Paré, his student Guillemeau, and Mauriceau had condemned this operation. Mauriceau claimed that, women's gossip to the contrary notwithstanding, no woman had survived the operation. How are we to imagine it?

In 1766, Jean Astruc claimed that it was possible to save the lives of both mother and child, citing M. Simon, surgeon at Saint-Cosme who published sixty-four case histories on the possible success of Caesarian section, and M. Soumain, qualified surgeon of Paris, who in 1740 successfully performed a Caesarian section in the presence of several of his colleagues.[79] Nontheless, not until the publication of Baudeloque's work at the end of the century did precise technical details about symphysis of the pubic bone and Caesarian section suggest that these operations were performed with any frequency. Before then one must think of surgical procedures as practiced exclusively on dead women. The criteria of what constitutes definitive death were not fully defined, and they remained a crucial question for the thinkers of the eighteenth century.[80] Surgical procedures in desperate cases, performed on living but exhausted, half-conscious, or crazed women, affected those who witnessed them as a scandalous, barbaric, and traumatic experience.

As the means of intervention became more circumscribed, a new passion for the "natural order of things" came into being, lending fuel to the eternal debate between the proponents of progress and active endeavor and the defenders of the natural processes. In the century of Rousseau, and involving as dramatic a problem as childbirth, the conflict became a confrontation of two schools. The matrons of village and neighborhood, excluded from any surgical training and held in contempt by the surgeons, were a powerful factor in keeping the terror of innovation alive in families. It was widely thought that if the forceps was used the child would die and the mother would be unable to have any more children. The obstetricians had great difficulties in obtaining the consent of families, midwives, and old physicians.[81]

Until the last years of the eighteenth century, the reaction against any surgical technique was intense. Citoyen Sacombe, who founded the anti-Caesarean school of Paris in 1799, bears witness to the views of a traditional but passionate elite: "The art of obstetrics has become a mere craft, relegated to the category of the mechanical arts."[82] Sacombe outlined the organization of a school into groups of twenty students, sponsored public debates with the "Baudeloquistes," and promised to conduct a formal experiment in which he would deliver a woman with a misshapen pelvis whose case would be considered hopeless by his colleagues. The pamphlets of the anti-Caesarean school accused Baudeloque, Dubois, and their likes of murdering and disemboweling pregnant women. Such excitement was uncalled for, yet it obviously expressed the dominant mentality and the collective terror in the face of suffering inflicted by the hand of man rather than willed by God. "By his case studies of the Year II, the founder of this school has loyally and solemnly challenged all wielders of instruments and hooks, all performers of Cesarian and symphytic sections to carry out all deliveries by hand. Are we living in the sixteenth or in the eighteenth century; are we among the French or among the canibals? I call upon the ghosts of the Baillys, the Rouchers, the Lavoisiers to come to our defense!"[83]

The men and women of the seventeenth and eighteenth centuries experienced childbirth as a phenomenon over which they had no control. The risk involved in giving birth is visible in psychological and demographic facts. The few pages of this essay have attempted to develop this theme under three of its aspects: collective ignorance, suffering and death, and the filtering down of progress. In each of these areas, some things are clear and some give rise to more questions: What can we know? What remains obscure? What are the possible directions of further research?

The ignorance of the matrons and of the women in childbirth themselves was not fortuitous. The elite of the practitioners, who used a concrete language and made their experiences known to a wider public, ran counter to an age-old mental block. There is concrete evidence that the men of the eighteenth century mounted considerable resistance to realistic research, mechanist terminology, and the use of new tools. (It was particularly strong since these tools were made of metal. Resistance of this kind is also encountered in black societies of Central Africa, for wood is a God-given material, while metal is forged by man and charged with notions of impurity.) The overwhelming majority of midwives and surgeon-barbers lived by an ancestral body of knowledge, unwilling to consider new practices, and the women in childbirth were passive and dominated. Superstition and guilt functioned as a mask disguising ignorance and anxiety. The explanations I have spontaneously advanced—modesty, religiously motivated contempt for physical life, sexual interdicts, great value attached to sacrifice, fear of life in general—are overly cursory. They should be reconsidered as elements of a vast mental heritage, which may well bring out the meaning of traditions handed down through the generations or of the humble experience of the individual.

Just as we do not have any document showing how a midwife accused of ignorance and absurd behavior would explain and defend herself, so all of our information concerning the painful and tragic side of childbirth comes from the outside. Eyewitness accounts show the woman in childbirth reaching a threshold of pain that makes her lose control of herself: convulsions, fainting, hysteria, fever, fatal hemorrhaging. But in the absence of firsthand testimony, we know very little (for the eyewitness accounts are primarily concerned with the unusual and the dramatic). The parish registers, long series of which are yet to be examined, will furnish figures for mortality in childbirth as well as very approximate figures for the mortality of newborn infants, since stillborn, and especially premature, infants were not listed. As for the aftereffects of difficult deliveries or violent manipulations, they have left no written trace at all. No historian will be able to quantify these infirmities, for they were never described by the physician and were borne by the women in silence and shame.

We should also try to assess the aftereffects for the child of unwanted pregnancy, attempted abortion, a long drawn-out delivery, and fear. And what was the proportion of children born deformed or misshapen? In our own day, we are beginning to recognize the influence of the few hours of birth on a child's physical and mental future.[84] In the past, more than now, maimed and defective children were part of one's familiar environment in village and neighborhood. Our ignorance of the objective facts is great, as is our unfamiliarity with the sensibility of the people of the past. We feel that we are living in a tragic universe; to what extent were experiences that to us would constitute an outrage of pain and insecurity borne by the women of the old society with an equanimity that we would consider fatalistic? It is important to reconstitute—as historians of death such as F. Lebrun and M. Vovelle have done—the emotional universe of the people of the past. Constantly living with threats of one kind or another, accustomed to hunger and suffering, familiar with early death, and imbued with the importance of duty accomplished, they may well have been obliged to develop a kind of serenity in the face of their own and their children's destiny.

And finally, how can we discern whether any progress was made in the day-to-day practice of midwifery and whether a change of attitudes took place in the last years of the Ancien Régime? The proliferation of manuals, the efforts to disseminate a body of knowledge and to regulate the profession of midwife are undeniable facts of the eighteenth century. Yet an appreciable decline of mortality in childbirth becomes clearly discernible only in subsequent centuries. Obstetrics could not evolve in isolation. Now that the advances in medicine of the nineteenth and twentieth centuries have led to the gradual disappearance of generalized infection and the various forms of hemorrhage, it will be possible to approach the problems of childbirth in different terms. The dissemination of knowledge in the eighteenth century marked an important stage, but by comparison with the unchanged pattern of practices and behaviors, it was but a surface wave.

NOTES

1. One of the principal themes in the work of Margaret Mead and Niles Newton on childbirth and motherhood is their universal ritualization. See "Conception, Pregnancy, Labor, and the Puerperium," in *First International Congress of Psychosomatic Medicine and Childbirth* (Paris, 1965), pp. 51-54.

2. To cite only the most recent studies: J. T. Noonan, *Contraception: A History of Its Treatment by the Catholic Theologians and Canonists* (Cambridge, Mass., 1965): J. Dupâquier and M. Lachiver, "Sur les débuts de la contraception en France ou les deux malthusianismes," *Annales, E.S.C.* 24 (November-December 1969): 1391-1406; J. L. Flandrin, *L'Eglise et le contrôle des naissances* (Paris, 1970); A. Lottin, "Naissances illégitimes et les filles-mères à Lille au XVIIIe siècle," *Revue d'histoire moderne et contemporaine* 17 (April-June 1970): 278-322; J.-L. Flandrin, "La Cellule familiale et l'oeuvre de procréation dans l'ancienne société," *Revue du XVIIe siècle* (1972); F. Lebrun, "Naissances illégitimes et abandons d'enfants en Anjou au XVIIIe siècle," *Annales, E.S.C.* 27 (July-October 1972): 1183-89; M. Laget, "Abandons d'enfants et troubles populaires à Narbonne (XVII-XVIIIes siècles)," in *Actes du Congrès de la Fédération historique du Languedoc-Rousillon* (Montpellier, 1973); series of articles on the French population in the seventeenth and eighteenth century published in J. Dupâquier, ed., *Hommages à Marcel Reinhard* (Paris, 1973); "Enfant et Société," special issue of *Annales de démographie historique* (1973).

3. L. Chertok et al., *Fémininité et maternité* (Paris, 1966), p. 45.

4. G.-L. Engelmann, *La Pratique des accouchements chez les peuples primitifs* (Paris, 1885), p. 15.

5. François Mauriceau, *Traité des maladies des femmes grosses et de celles qui sont accouchées* (Paris, Latin edition of 1668, 7 editions until 1740).

6. J.-L. Baudelocque, *L'Art des accouchements*, 2 vols. (Paris, 1796).

7. Jean-Noël Biraben, "Le Médecin et l'enfant au XVIIIe siècle: Aperçu sur la pédiatrie," *Annales de démographie historique* (1973): p. 215.

8. Philippe Peu, *La Pratique des accouchements* (Paris, 1694).

9. Mme. Le Boursier du Coudray, mistress of midwifery, *Abrégé de l'art des accouchemens* (Paris, 1769).

10. J. Mesnard, *Le Guide des accoucheurs* (Paris, 1753).

11. Emmanuel Le Roy Ladurie, "Démographie et funestes secrets," *Annales historiques de la Révolution française* 37 (1965): 385-400.

12. See, in particular, J.-M. Gouesse, "En basse Normandie aux XVIIe et XVIIIe siècles: Le Refus de l'enfant au tribunal de la pénitence," *Annales de démographie historique* (1973).

13. Flandrin, *L'Eglise et le contrôle des naissances,* p. 8.

14. Le Roy Ladurie, "Funestes secrets."

15. J.-P. Gutton, *La Société et les pauvres: L'Exemple de la généralité de Lyon* (Paris, 1971), p. 65.

16. Philippe Ariès, "Attitudes devant la vie et devant la mort du XVII au XIXe siècle," *Population* 4 (1949): 463-70.

17. A Molinier, "Enfants trouvés, enfants abandonés, enfants illégitimes en Languedoc aux XVIIe et XVIIIe siècles," in *Hommages à Marcel Reinhard.*

18. Nicolas Puzos, *Traité des accouchements* (Paris, 1759).

19. B. Malinowski, *La Sexualité, sa répression dans les sociétés primitives* (Paris, 1967).

20. See, in particular, J.-L. Flandrin, "L'Attitude à légard du petit enfant et les conduites sexuelles dans la civilisation occidentale," *Annales de démographie historique* (1973): pp. 143-210.

21. Philippe Ariès, *L'Enfant et la vie familiale sous l'Ancien Régime,* 2d ed. (Paris, 1972), preface, p. ix (English translation by Robert Baldick, *Centuries of Childhood* [New York, 1962]).

22. A. Bideau, "L'Envoi de jeunes enfants en nourrice (Thoissey-en-Dombes, 1740-1780)," in *Hommages à Marcel Reinhard.*

23. See Archives départementales [hereafter A.D.], Hérault, D 178, M. Rigail, *Dissertation sur l'asphyxie des enfants naissant où l'on rapporte un nouveau moyen de les rappeler à la vie.*

24. Michel Raulin, *Instructions succinctes sur les accouchements en faveur des sages-femmes des provinces* (Paris, 1770), pp. 18 ff.

25. Ariès, *L'Enfant et la vie familiale,* preface, p. ix.

26. A.D., Hérault, G 432.

27. See M. Laget, "Recherches sur les ondoiements et baptêmes à Lodève et dans son diocèse aux XVIIe et XVIIIe siècles," *Etudes sur Pézenas et sa région* 6, no. 3 (1975).

28. Georges Witowski, *Accoucheurs et sages-femmes célèbres* (Paris, 1887).

29. Bernadette Bonnet, "Etude obstétricale sur le rituel de l'accouchement à propos de quelques sociétés primitives" (Thesis in medicine, University of Paris, 1972).

30. C. Revault d'Allonnes, "La Douleur et l'indolorisation psychologique des accouchements" (Thesis, University of Paris, 1971).

31. Engelmann, *La Pratique des accouchements.*

32. Niles Newton, "Certains aspects de l'accouchement chez les peuples primitifs," *Vie médicale,* special issue (Christmas, 1965).

33. Puzos, *Traité des accouchements.*

34. See below.

35. Revault Allones, "La Douleur."

36. "Last burden, called thus because it truly is the second burden the pregnant woman sheds in her confinement after she has shed the first burden, which is the child. It is also called placenta, that is, pie or cake, because that is what it resembles. It is rightly called *délivre,* since it ends the delivery of the woman in labor" Peu, (*La Pratique,* p. 34).

37. See below.

38. Text edited at Montpellier in 1873 with an introduction by Elie Fraisse.

39. A.D., Hérault, D 179, M. Rigail, *Mémoire sur les accouchements.*

40. Puzos, *Traité des accouchements.*

41. G.-J. Engelmann; *De l'accouchement comparé dans les races humaines* (Paris: Savy, 1885), 11 pp.

42. G.-R. Lefebvre de Saint Ildefont, *Le Manuel des femmes enceintes, de celles qui sont en couches, et des mères qui veulent nourrir* (Paris. 1777).

43. A.D., Hérault, D 179.

44. Claude Lévi-Strauss, *Anthropologie structurale* (Paris, 1958), pp. 205 ff.

45. F. Doublet, *Nouvelles recherches sur la fièvre puerpérale* (Paris, 1791).

46. René Baudart, "Considérations sur les formes graves de l'infection puerpérale" (Thesis in medicine, University of Paris, 1936).

47. Jean-Baptiste Demangeon, *Examen critique de la doctrine et des procédés du citoyen Sacombe* (Paris, 1800).

48. A.D., Hérault, Clermont l'Hérault (GG 12, GG 13, GG 16); Maugio (GG 2, GG 3, GG 7); Montpellier (3 E 177^9 and 177^{13}); Municipal Archives of Montpellier, registers of Sainte-Anne parish, 1750-53.

49. Bonnet, *Etude obstétricale.*

50. Philippe Hecquet, *De l'indécence aux hommes d'accoucher les femmes* (Trévoux, 1708).

51. G. de la Motte, *Dissertation sur la génération. Réponse au livre: "De l'indécence aux hommes d'accoucher les femmes"* (Paris, 1718).

52. Elisabeth Nihell, *Traité sur les accouchements par les femmes* (Paris, 1771).

53. Witowski, in *Accoucheurs et sages-femmes célèbres,* cites many midwives, especially those of the Hotel-Dieu between 1601 and 1774.

54. Louise Bourgeois, *Instructions à ma fille* (Paris, 1626).

55. Marguerite de la Marche, *Instructions familières et très faciles par questions et réponses touchant toutes les choses principales qu'une sage-femme doit savoir* (Paris, 1626).

56. Le Boursier du Coudray, *Abrégé de l'art des accouchements.*

57. See below.

58. "The choice of the women that were sent to these courses was not made carefully enough. Since most of them, indeed two thirds or one half, cannot read and do not understand French, how could one hope that they would understand the jargon of the art? All that these women have brought back from traveling to the capitals is a great deal of boldness and an insolent but dangerous self-assurance" (M. Nicolas, *Le Cri de la nature en faveur des enfants nouveau-nés* [Paris, 1775]).

59. See below.

60. Mauriceau, *Traité.*

61. Ibid.

62. Peu, *La Pratique.*

63. J. Matthieu, *Les Accoucheuses traditionnelles de Casablanca* (Paris, 1952).

64. Raulin, *Instructions,* introduction, p. iv.

65. J. Manicom, *La Graine: Journal d'une sage-femme* (Paris, 1973), pp. 183 ff.

66. A. D., Hérault, C 2776, *Enquête sur les chirurgiens et les sages-femmes de la province de Languedoc, 1737;* C 525, *Enquête sur les sages-femmes de la province de Languedoc, 1786.*

67. Archives communales de Sète, B B 1172.

68. A.D., Hérault, G 1172, *Enquêtes diocisaines de 1684 et 1689.*

69. Ibid., G 1163 (1698-99).

70. Ibid., 100 M 1, 100 M 2 (1806-10).

71. F. Furet and W. Sachs, "La Croissance de l'alphabétisation en France (XVIII-XIX

siècle)," *Annales, E.S.C.* 29 (May-June 1974): 714-37.

72. P. Amand, *Questions générales sur les accouchements* (Paris, 1713).

73. P. Augier du Fot, *Catéchisme de l'art des accouchements* (Montpellier, 1776).

74. P. Delmas, *Sept siècles d'obstétrique à la faculté de médecine de Montpellier* (Montpellier, 1927).

75. The difficult personality of Sénaux, who was constantly fighting with the faculty of medicine and the minister Chaptal and the interminable discussions about the projected building of a school of midwifery within the walls of the hospice make the bundles 100 M 14-100 M 17 of the departmental archives of Hérault interesting reading indeed. Sénaux's many proposals, the transfer of materials from the faculty of medicine, the organization of courses, and the concept of obstetrical teaching connected with the daily life of a hospice may become the subject of a later study.

76. Cited by M. Fosseyeux, "Sages-femmes et nourrices à Paris au XVIIe siècle," *Revue de Paris* (1921), pp. 535-54.

77. Cited by P. Costet, "De l'extraction de la tête dernière (manoeuvre de Mauriceau)" (Thesis of medicine, University of Paris, 1935).

78. See Biraben, "Le Médecin," p. 215.

79. Jean Astruc, *L'Art d'accoucher réduit à ses principes* (Paris, 1766), pp. 293-318.

80. A.D., Hérault, D 178, M. Rigail, *Mémoire sur l'opération césarienne pratiquée sur une femme morte.*

81. Jean-Baptiste Demangeon, *Le Jeune Médecin vis-à-vis du vieux* (Paris, an XII [1804]).

82. Citoyen Sacombe, *Les Douze Mois de l'école anti-césarienne* (Paris, 1799).

83. Ibid., p. 56.

84. See F. Leboyer, *Pour une naissance sans violence* (Paris, 1974); English translation, *Birth without Violence* (New York, 1975).